W9-CQC-268

inside
weight lifting
and weight training

inside
weight lifting
and weight training

jim murray

cbi **Contemporary Books, Inc.**
Chicago

Library of Congress Cataloging in Publication Data

Murray, Jim.
   Inside weight lifting and weight training.

   Bibliography: p.
   Includes index.
   1. Weight lifting. 2. Physical fitness.
I. Title.
GV546.M85   796.4'1   77-75844
ISBN 0-8092-7806-5
ISBN 0-8092-7805·7 pbk.

Copyright © 1977 by Jim Murray
All rights reserved.
Published by Contemporary Books, Inc.
180 North Michigan Avenue, Chicago, Illinois 60601
Manufactured in the United States of America
Library of Congress Catalog Card Number: 77-75844
International Standard Book Number: 0-8092-7806-5 (cloth)
                         0-8092-7805-7 (paper)

Published simultaneously in Canada by
Beaverbooks
953 Dillingham Road
Pickering, Ontario L1W 1Z7
Canada

contents

acknowledgments

I want to thank my wife, Jane, for her encouragement and for helping with the typing; June Ludwig for her able assistance with the typing; Bob Cappiello and my sons, Jim III and Jay, for demonstrating the exercises; T. J. Klein for taking the posed exercise photos; Bruce Klemens for the action pictures of weight-lifting competition; and John Grimek for lending the snapshot proving that muscles, once developed, can last a lifetime. The photo of John lifting, taken in 1940, was originally published in *Strength & Health* magazine.

INTRODUCTION

How fast can you run? How far can you throw? How high can you jump? How much can you lift?

These are the elemental questions that are answered by performance in athletic sports. Such basic abilities are the primitive qualities that once were necessary to survival; so it is not surprising that performances calling for power, strength, and speed continue to fascinate most people.

Few qualities are more intriguing than strength—or power, which is strength with speed. And nothing provides a better measurement of strength and power than lifting weights, for the implement used—a barbell —is standardized, and the weights are the same everywhere, whether they are measured in pounds or kilograms.

It is true that skill can be a factor in lifting weights. And it is also true that some people have structural advantages that make them better suited to lifting than others. But setting such facts as these aside, it takes a very strong man to lift 200 pounds overhead, a stronger one to lift 250 to 300 pounds, and an absolutely superstrong one to lift more than 300 pounds.

The difficulty in lifting from 200 to 300 pounds overhead became evident to large numbers of people when the ''Superstars'' competition was televised nationally and it could be seen that very few champion athletes, including many who used weight training in their conditioning programs, were able to lift such heavy weights. Only physical giants such as professional football players, shot-putters, and Mr. Universe winners were able to lift weights in the 250- to 300-pound range overhead.

In fact, it takes a good measure of strength just to lift 200 or 300 pounds a few inches off the floor. How, then, can we describe in words the incredible power of a champion weight lifter as he raises 500 pounds from the floor to his chest in a clean and then proceeds to ram the weight overhead?

We can gain some insight into the magnitude of a 500-pound lift overhead by comparing it to the four-minute mile, a great milestone in measurable athletic performance. It was in 1954 that Roger Bannister first ran a mile in slightly under four minutes, actually 3:59.4. During the same year, heavyweight champion Norbert Schemansky set a world weight lifting record by cleaning and jerking 425 pounds. Schemansky had become the first weight lifter who was "comfortable" with 400 pounds or more, though Charles Rigoulot and John Davis had previously broken the 400-pound barrier, each with a lift of 402 pounds.

Twenty-one years after Bannister showed it could be done, John Walker ran a mile in 3:49.4, just 10 seconds faster than Bannister's breakthrough effort. That same year, 1975, Vasily Alexeyev, the 345-pound Russian superheavyweight, raised a record 545½ pounds in the clean and jerk. While the efforts of myriad runners were chipping away to a four percent improvement in the record for the mile, the weight lifting record had been improved by a whopping 28 percent!

WEIGHT LIFTING AND WEIGHT TRAINING

It is important to understand the difference between weight lifting and weight training, which many people think of as the same thing. Actually, the two are inseparable because, in their simplest form, they consist of pulling and pushing against graded resistance in the form of a barbell. (A barbell consists of a steel bar and iron disks, or plates, of various weights. The bar serves as a handle to be gripped. The plates are slipped onto each end of the bar by means of holes at their centers.)

The essential difference between weight lifting and weight training is that the former is a standardized international sport—practiced more widely throughout the world than the familiar Amcrican sports of football and baseball—requiring skill as well as great strength. Weight training is a basic form of exercise that is needed by anyone—athlete or nonathlete—who wants to develop a full

measure of strength, look his or her best, and enjoy the pleasant kinesthetic sensation of having superior physical fitness.

The value of the weight training described in this book is well established. The book is a distillation of more than thirty years of practical experience and study and also draws on the knowledge and experience of educators, scientists, and champion athletes who have contributed to better understanding of exercise over the past century. There is more to learn about weight training and weight lifting than this book can teach, and the section on competitive lifting can be considered only an introduction to the sport and a basic reference, but the section on weight training provides as much as anyone needs to know in order to use the activity to develop and maintain superior general strength and physical fitness. In addition the weight training described not only can serve as an introduction to competitive weight lifting, but also can provide a beginner with the early groundwork preliminary to specializing in bodybuilding or another type of strength competition called power lifting. More detailed information on bodybuilding and power lifting can be obtained from the books on bodybuilding by Franco Columbu and on power lifting by Terry Todd, both published by Contemporary Books, Inc.

Actually, the use of weight training to develop strength and weight lifting to demonstrate it predate recorded history. Legend tells the story of Milo, an athlete of ancient Greece, who developed his strength by lifting and carrying a young bull every day until it reached maturity. As the bull grew in weight, Milo's muscles adapted by growing in strength, until finally he became an Olympic champion in the form of modified mayhem that passed for wrestling in those bygone days.

The modern principle of weight training is the same: regular exercise against progressively increasing resistance. Instead of shouldering a mass of quivering and perhaps protesting live weight, however, the modern strength athlete or fitness seeker has the convenience of a machined barbell handle, knurled to assist his grip, and he can vary the amount of weight he exercises with by adding or subtracting balanced plates at the ends of the handles.

In weight training (and competitive lifting, for that matter), you begin with an amount of weight that is easy to lift so you can learn to perform the exercise properly. At the same time, you experiment to determine the amount of weight you can use while performing a given number of repetitions of an exercise. The recommended approach is to begin with a weight you can lift for five to eight repetitions, continuing to use the same amount of weight each time you exercise, while attempting to add one or two repetitions at each exercise session. When you can perform ten, twelve, or fifteen repetitions, add enough weight to restrict the repetitions to five or eight and begin the progression again. The muscles are coaxed along, adapting to this gradually increasing challenge by becoming stronger and, to some extent, larger.

inside
weight lifting
and weight training

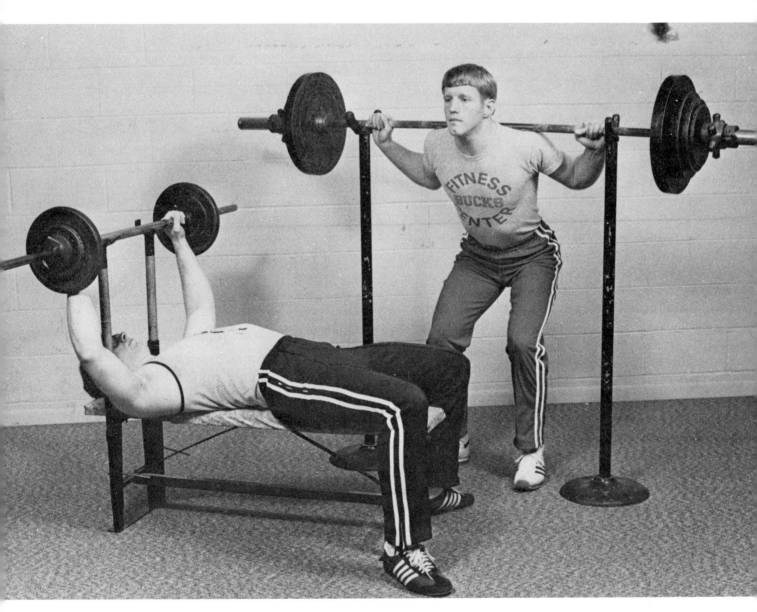

Fig. 1. The photo shows essential items of equipment used in weight training: a bench, with uprights, for the supine press exercise, and a pair of shoulder-high stands. The barbell on the bench is a typical exercise set, and the one on the stands is a revolving competition set, used for Olympic lifting.

chapter 1

BEGINNING WEIGHT TRAINING

To begin a weight training program—which is preliminary to various kinds of competition as well as a fitness-building end in itself—you need access to a barbell. Ideally, you might join a gymnasium or health club where weights, instruction, training partners, and accessory equipment are available. But you can begin alone and at home. Here's how. First purchase a basic barbell set, preferably one that includes short dumbbell handles and at least four 10-pound, four 5-pound, four 2½-pound, and four 1¼-pound plates. The reason it is important to get these smaller plates in fours is that they can be used on the dumbbells for some important shoulder-strengthening exercises. If you are in normal health, male, and of reasonably average size, there is no point in starting with anything smaller than a 100-pound adjustable barbell. The assortment of plates listed above adds up to 75 pounds. A five-foot steel barbell handle weighs 15 pounds and the usual set of inside and outside collars used to hold the plates in place brings the total weight to 100 pounds. (These are usually called 110-pound

combination sets, but that is the shipping weight, including the weights of the dumbbell bars and collars.)

One hundred pounds is enough weight for a keep-fit program for anyone, yet not too light to begin with should you become serious about developing superior strength. Iron plates are preferable to plastic because they take up less space on the bar and leave room for any large plates that you may decide to purchase later.

A person who wants to develop and maintain superior physical fitness can do so with no equipment other than a barbell (for strength) and a pair of jogging shoes (for cardiorespiratory conditioning). But to progress beyond the most elementary stage of strength training, you also need a bench designed specifically for the supine press exercise and a pair of supports from which you can take a barbell across your shoulders with a partial bend of your knees. Fig. 1 shows these items of basic equipment. A 110-pound barbell/dumbbell combination set with iron plates may cost forty to fifty dollars, an exercise bench with upright supports for supine pressing about forty dollars, and supports used for shouldering a heavy weight about forty to fifty dollars. These items are good investments because they are practically indestructible and with reasonable care will last more than a lifetime.

Beyond this basic equipment, you can buy additional barbell plates for about thirty-five to fifty cents a pound. Thus a 100-pound barbell set becomes a 200-pound set with the purchase of a pair of 50-pound plates. This investment, and more, will be necessary for the serious home exerciser because an average-sized young man of 140 to 160 pounds can develop enough strength to perform leg exercises with 200 pounds in a few months' time.

Another worthwhile investment for serious home exercisers is a six-foot bar, which costs about fifteen dollars. Most exercise sets are sold with five-foot barbell handles, and these are too short to accommodate heavier poundages. With a six-foot barbell handle, you can place the inside collars as far as 48 inches apart and still leave enough room at the ends for heavy loads of plates, especially if you have 50- and 25-pound plates. These weights and the longer bar will be required if you want to try the competition lifts, described later, with an exercise set. The alternative is to obtain an Olympic standard barbell, which is the ideal lifting implement but is so expensive that most such sets are found in clubs and various kinds of public gymnasiums. A 300-pound Olympic set costs more than $250 and a 400-pound set more than $300. An Olympic set is an excellent investment, however, for unlike most recreational and sporting equipment, it never really wears out. The Olympic barbell will be described in more detail in the section devoted to competitive lifting.

WHAT HAPPENS WHEN YOU LIFT WEIGHTS?

Weight lifting has a complex effect on the body, and this book will not attempt to go into all the physiological and kinesiological details. A basic idea of what happens should be of interest, however, and the essence of it is as follows. When the body is subjected to a stress, it attempts to adapt and compensate so that when a similar stress occurs, it can be handled more easily. When the muscles and skeletal structures are stressed by lifting a weight, the body compensates by becoming stronger.

The muscles, which consist of many tiny contractile fibers, do not push; they exert force by contracting, or shortening. When you push against something with your arms or legs, the muscles that provide the impetus work by shortening to extend the levers that are your bones. The idea of muscles working by shortening is easy to grasp when you think of raising a weight from your side to your shoulder by flexing (bending) your arm. Obviously, the biceps muscle along the front of your arm is contracting into a lump. Similar contractions of other muscles occur if you then proceed to push the weight up over your head. For you to push something upward, the deltoid muscle of your shoulder must contract to raise your arm, and the final bit of push that straightens your arm upward comes from the contracting pull of the triceps muscle along the back of your arm.

It is worth noting that when you perform exercises for opposing muscles—the muscles that flex the arm, for example, and the muscles that extend the arm—the muscles that are not contracting are relaxing and being stretched. Therefore, you have no reason to worry that exercising with weights will "shorten" a muscle and restrict its range of motion, as long as the opposing muscles are also exercised.

Within the muscles themselves a highly complicated process is underway. When the muscle fibers are challenged by being called upon to work against substantial resistance, there is an increase of a substance called actomyosin, which makes the fibers stronger and somewhat thicker. When the muscles are worked against minimal resistance, so little force is required to overcome it and the exercise can be repeated many times, the muscles respond by increasing a material called sarcoplasm more than by building up actomyosin.

Sarcoplasm is produced by repetitive, low-force activity such as running, whereas the brief, high-force activity of weight lifting produces actomyosin. Therefore, sarcoplasm is associated with muscular endurance and actomyosin with muscular strength. To some extent, training for endurance handicaps strength and training for strength handicaps endurance. This is most evident when extreme performance is the goal. A marathon runner must run long distances to train for his event; if he trains as a weight lifter does and neglects running, he will be poorly prepared for his kind of competition. A weight lifter must train with heavy weights in brief bursts; if he spends a great deal of time running, his strength will suffer.

Brian Oldfield, the 6' 5", 270-pound superathlete who became the first man to put the 16-pound shot 75 feet, commented that intensive endurance training adversely affected his strength. In an interview by Garry Hill, published in *Track & Field News,* Oldfield said he had prepared for the television ''Superstars'' competition by training for swimming and bicycling with the result that his strength dissipated. As his bench press dropped from 400 to 300 pounds, his ability to put the shot suffered. In retrospect, he said, ''I just should have stayed with my weight training and I would have been stronger in all the [''Superstars''] events. All I ended up doing was breaking down muscle fiber.'' Incidentally, despite the fact that he felt the endurance work had broken down muscle fiber, Oldfield did win the weight lifting by hoisting 300 and 310 pounds overhead, lifts that were considerably less than his best when he trained primarily for strength.

Although great emphasis on either strength or endurance training has an adverse effect on the quality that is not emphasized, the experience of champion athletes suggests that a certain amount of strength training improves the performance of those in endurance events and that a certain amount of endurance work, such as jogging, improves the performance of those in events requiring strength and power. Many champion runners include some weight training in their training programs, and many champions in such power sports as weight lifting and shot-putting do some running.

The value of combined training is especially evident in the careers of athletes successful in events requiring both strength and endurance. One is Dan Gable, the Olympic wrestling champion, who did a great deal of running for endurance and weight training for strength. Another is Olympic decathlon champion Bruce Jenner, who mixed weight training for strength and power with the running required for the track events of his ten-event specialty.

On a basis of the experience of champion athletes and other more ordinary people who have exercised with weights for many years, we know that a good general approach to weight training is to work with a resistance that permits an intermediate number of repetitions, in the range of five to ten. This tends to produce both muscular strength and endurance. There is another advantage to working with a resistance that permits at least five repetitions: it is safer. You are much less likely to strain or ''pull'' a muscle with a weight you can lift five times than with a weight you can lift only once with an all-out effort.

To develop great strength and explosive power, however, you must at least occasionally work with weights that require an all-out effort for only one to three lifts. This is a ''must'' in the training of champion lifters and is also practiced by most athletes who use weight training in preparation for sports that require explosive power, such as shot-putting and high jumping.

An example of a shot-putter who trained with very heavy weights in explosive movements is Al Feuerbach, who won the United States AAU heavyweight (242-pound class) weight lifting championship the same year that he broke the world shot put record with distances of more than 70 feet. Feuerbach could clean and jerk well over 400 pounds. Less well known is the fact that high jumper Dwight Stones also practiced explosive weight lifting exercises, such as the clean and jerk, to help develop the power to high jump at world record 7½-foot levels. To prepare for his assaults on the high jump record, the 6′5″, 178-pound Stones worked up from 135 to as much as 220 pounds in the clean and jerk. He used the same weights, performing more repetitions, for squats with a barbell on his shoulders.

It is instructive, too, to note that weight training had different effects on Feuerbach and Stones, even though each lifted as much as he was able. Feuerbach, who had heavy bones and a sturdy structure, developed massive muscles. Stones's lighter natural structure limited his gain in bulk, and the primary result of his training was a gain in strength and power: he became very strong for his physical type.

THE EFFECT OF THE SOMATOTYPE

An individual's response to weight training —or to any type of exercise, for that matter —depends a great deal on genetic endowment. To a certain extent, champions are "made," but it is also true that champions are "born." A naturally short, stocky person may practice basketball for hours but never become a star basketball player. A tall, rangy, small-boned person may practice weight lifting but is unlikely to become a champion in the sport.

The reason that the tall high jumper develops strength and power without much increase in size is that his *somatotype*, or body type, is highly ectomorphic. The reason that the shot-putter develops massive muscles from much the same kind of exercise is that his somatotype is predominantly mesomorphic.

It is worth digressing for a moment to discuss somatotyping briefly, because your physical type has a great deal to do with how you respond to exercise. Somatotyping was developed by anthropologist William H. Sheldon, who rated the human physique according to three components: endomorphy, mesomorphy, and ectomorphy. Endomorphy is the roundness and fatness component, mesomorphy is the muscle and bone component, and ectomorphy is the leanness and fragility component. Sheldon rated people on a scale of one to seven for each of these three qualities and considered that no one, however extreme his physical type, would rate a zero in any of them. According to his system, an extremely thin, narrow-shouldered, small-boned person with very little fat would have a 1-1-7 somatotype. A heavily muscled, wide-shouldered, large-boned person, also with little fat, would be a 1-7-1. And a soft, pear-shaped person with little muscle and a lot of fat would be a 7-1-1.

Few people have such pure somatotypes as to rate seven in one component and only one in each of the others. It is easy to see that a shot-putter like Feuerbach rates at the highest levels of mesomorphy—perhaps seven; at least six. Stones, the high jumper, rates high in ectomorphy, but a closer look shows that there is also mesomorphy in his makeup, as evidenced by considerable muscular development. Athletes in vigorous sports may have a predominance of ectomorphy or a large endomorphic component, but they are seldom really low in mesomorphy. Alexeyev, the gigantic Russian superheavyweight lifter who was the first to clean and jerk 500 pounds, might seem essentially endomorphic to the casual observer of his protruding abdomen. But a closer look reveals the massive bone and muscle of the mesomorph. From the back, Alexeyev displays the wide-

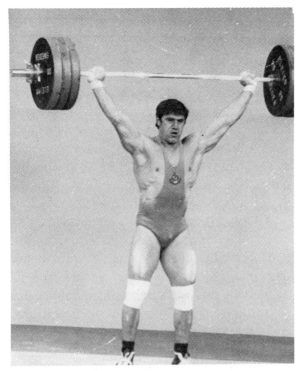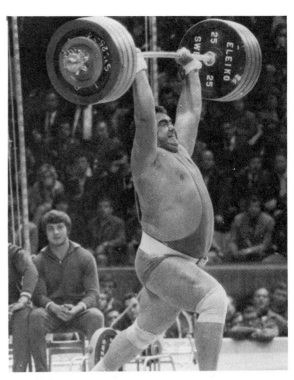

Figs. 2 and 3. The physiques of David Rigert, world 198-pound champion, and superheavyweight champ Vasily Alexeyev provide an interesting contrast. Both are highly mesomorphic, but the trim Rigert, at 5 feet 9½ inches and 198 pounds, is less endomorphic than the gigantic Alexeyev, who weighs 345 and stands slightly over 6 feet tall. Although Alexeyev lifts more weight—he is pictured holding 541 pounds—Rigert is a much better lifter in proportion to his size. He is shown holding 363 pounds with the typical wide grip used for the snatch.

shouldered, tapering-down appearance that is admired in a masculine physique. It is only when he is viewed from angles displaying his expansive midsection and double chin that the endomorphic part of his physical makeup is evident.

Most people have more intermediate somatotypes. Unless the mesomorphic component is very low, most men can anticipate a substantial increase in strength and some visible evidence of increased muscle size and change in muscle shape as a result of weight training. The greater the inherent mesomorphic component, the greater the potential for increased strength and muscle size. To some extent this is also true for women, but even a woman who is more mesomorphic than average will not become as strong and muscular as a similarly trained man, because she lacks male (androgenic) hormones. The effect of weight training on women is to make the muscles firmer and stronger and to improve shapeliness, but not to produce masculine-looking muscles.

NERVOUS SYSTEM LIMITS ON STRENGTH PERFORMANCE

Another thing that happens when you lift a weight—in fact, the first thing—is that your brain sends a message via the nervous system chain of command. The message is "interpreted" by the nervous system until ultimately—though in a split second's time—the small nerves that trigger contraction of individual muscle fibers respond so that just enough fibers contract to perform the amount of work that is called for. The fibers don't all contract at once, however, even in all-out efforts.

It is the limitation of the nervous system control that separates champions from also-rans. The champion has superior neuromuscular control. When his mind signals his muscles to lift, the final relays to the nerves that trigger contraction and relaxation are highly efficient, enabling him to get the most out of the effort. Theoretically, if a person had perfect control over his muscles, he could determine the absolute maximum amount he could lift one time in any given exercise and then obtain a complete muscular workout by lifting it once. This would be analogous to a high jumper reaching his best height in every practice and every competition, or to a baseball player hitting a home run every time a pitch was delivered into the strike zone.

Since no one has such perfect neuromuscular control, however, better results are obtained by lifting submaximal weights several times or, in the case of the competitive weight lifter, by performing several single lifts. During such repetitions, even the most inefficient nervous system activates different sets of fibers and you wind up having exercised the entire muscle effectively. In addition, repetitive exercises develop both the myofibrillar strength (actomyosin) and the endurance (sarcoplasm) components of the muscles. When the exercises are done in sets—that is, when each exercise is repeated several times and then, after a brief rest, done several times more—there is a superior conditioning effect.

CONDITIONING EFFECT OF WEIGHT TRAINING

Weight training is best used as one aspect of an overall conditioning program: the strength- and power-building part. When you perform several sets of a weight training exercise, however, there is also a demand on the heart and lungs. The activity uses up energy and therefore requires oxygen. As a result, you must breathe harder, and your heart must pump more vigorously to send oxygenated blood to the working muscles. An exercise such as cleaning a barbell from the floor to the chest, for example, brings all of the muscles of the body into play and requires a great deal of energy in a brief burst. When the ex-

ercise is repeated several times, the demand for oxygen is great, as it is in running a sprint race.

To meet the demand for oxygen, the heart rate increases, and the heart is believed to adapt to this demand by increasing the number and size of small blood vessels in its own muscle so that the same amount of work will be less stressful the next time it is encountered. The demand has a similar effect on blood vessels in the skeletal muscles.

Although your heart can't be tensed deliberately like your biceps, it is also a muscle and, like other muscles, can be strengthened and conditioned by exercise. There is general agreement among exercise physiologists that a "training effect" on the heart is achieved when the pulse rate rises to about seventy percent (sixty to eighty percent) of its maximum rate in response to physical activity. Your maximum rate decreases as you get older and is about 220 minus your age. At twenty to twenty-five years of age, seventy per cent of maximum would be 140 beats per minute. At thirty, it would be 136; at forty, 128; at forty-five, 124; at fifty, 119; at fifty-five, 115; at sixty, 111; and at sixty-five, 107. Maximums vary somewhat from one individual to another, and if you have any doubt about your fitness to exercise at the seventy percent-and-over level, you should have a medical examination first.

The best cardiovascular training effect is derived from such continuous activities as jogging, swimming, cycling, or rope skipping, but there is some general conditioning effect from regular weight training. If the rest between exercises is kept short, so that the heart rate does not return to its resting level, the general conditioning effect is increased. This fact is the basis for "circuit training" using weights, in which the exerciser performs an exercise for one body part, moves quickly to a second exercise for another body part, then to a third exercise, and so on until a circuit of perhaps ten exercises is completed. As the exerciser's strength and general condition improve, the circuit is

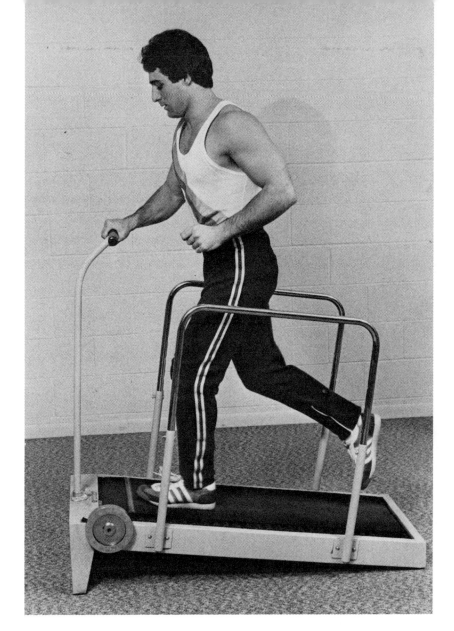

Fig. 4. Running or jogging is an effective way to exercise for cardiovascular fitness. Bob Cappiello is shown running on a treadmill, which is especially difficult because of the uphill slant.

speeded up, entire circuits are repeated several times, and rest periods between circuits are progressively shortened to make the workout ever more continuous.

For a general conditioning program giving major emphasis to strength, circuit training is very effective. It is most effective when part of the circuit is devoted to a brief bout of cardiovascular exercise, such as rope skipping or jumping jacks, and part is weight training exercises. But for really intensive strength work integrated with a cardiovascular program such as running, it is better to completely separate the two components of training. High levels of strength and power are best achieved by working against heavy resistance, and to work with heavy weights you must rest from one to three minutes be-

tween bouts of exercise. The more rest permitted between sets and exercises, the less cardiovascular training effect. Therefore, when training for strength at the relatively leisurely pace that is most effective, you should do your heart-and-lung conditioning separately. It will be less disturbing to your body if you do all your strength work before doing any endurance work such as running. If you run first, to put it in the simplest terms, you will be too "pooped" to do justice to the strength work. In fact, the best way to integrate strength and endurance programs in which you want to achieve relatively high levels of each is to do them on alternate days. In that way, you get adequate rest from the strength work for your body actually to build itself, and you get adequate

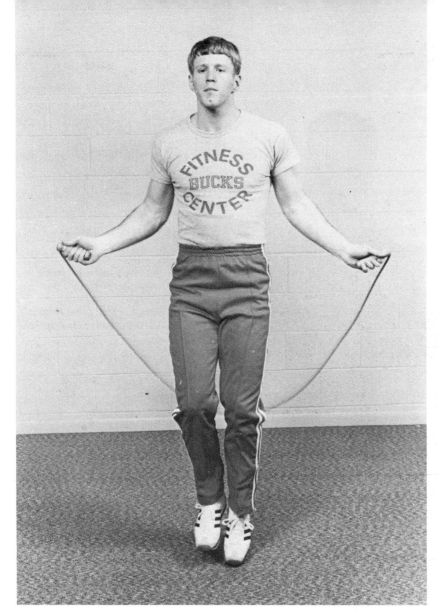

Fig. 5. A study seemed to show that ten minutes of rope skipping is equivalent in cardiovascular training effect to thirty minutes of jogging, but the study may actually have shown that ten minutes of such vigorous training is enough to produce aerobic benefit. The exercise is demonstrated by Jim Murray III, a former college football player who learned to skip rope while doing some amateur boxing.

(overnight) rest from the endurance training so that you can put a good effort into the strength program.

I don't mean to imply that a healthy individual can't adapt to both strength and endurance work on the same day. We see that it can be done whenever we watch a decathlon competition or wrestlers in action. But when endurance work is integrated with strength training in this manner, there is always a compromise. Neither strength nor endurance performance reaches its full potential. A program that handicaps strength and power is certainly not suitable for a shot-putter or a weight lifter, nor is a program that strongly emphasizes power training suitable for a distance runner.

A mixed program can be planned to include weight training on certain days and endurance exercises such as running or rope skipping on other days. The overall program can be set up to emphasize either strength or endurance. For example, weight training Monday-Wednesday-Friday and jogging Tuesday-Thursday emphasizes strength while providing some general cardiovascular conditioning. On the other hand, jogging and running Monday-Tuesday-Thursday-Friday and lifting Wednesday-Saturday emphasizes cardiovascular fitness while providing adequate strength and muscle tone.

Some studies of the physiology of exercise suggest that you obtain a cardiovascular training effect if you increase your heart rate briefly to a rate of at least 140 beats per minute, but many exercise physiologists believe you need to keep the rate at seventy percent of maximum continuously for at least ten to twenty minutes for a good training effect. Since ten minutes of rope skipping has been found equivalent to thirty minutes of jogging in producing a cardiovascular training effect, it is quite likely that the minimum effective dose of exercise hasn't yet been determined. In any event, this sustained elevated heart rate is accomplished much more efficiently with running than with weight training, which is why it is advisable to include both types of exercise in a general conditioning program rather than try to devise endurance programs with weights. Also, if you try to do serious endurance work with weights, you will have to keep the weight so light that your gains in strength will be handicapped.

EFFECT OF WEIGHT TRAINING ON HEALTH

There is a tendency to categorize weight training as beneficial to muscular strength, but as having little other positive benefit to health. Actually, few scientific investigators have looked for health benefits as a result of weight training and, in fact, some seem to be prejudiced against the activity without even attempting to understand it. Many scientists, like many laymen, seem to think the end result of weight training is either an extremely muscular Mr. America-type physique or a strong but somewhat fat body like those of the lifting champions in the unlimited weight class. Most people, scientists and laymen alike, will express admiration for the physique of an all-around athlete who succeeds in the decathlon—but these people do not realize that almost all decathlon champions are products of intensive weight training as well as of the running and jumping practice required in their sport. The 1976 Olympic decathlon champion and record setter, Bruce Jenner, said about one-third of his training consisted of weight training. The 1968 Olympic decathlon champion, Bill Toomey, who weighed about 190, could bench press more than 300 pounds.

At least part of the bias against muscles probably stems from a sour grapes attitude. Unfortunately, this bias has prompted many scientists to seek deficiencies associated with muscular development rather than to objectively try to determine whether there are any benefits other than strength from muscle-building exercise. At one time it was an "established fact" that muscle-building exercise would make its practitioner slow. It was also "well known" that weight lifting was dangerous and led to injuries. These two beliefs were proved fallacious by the late Dr. Peter Karpovich, research physiologist. He found that weight lifters could move their heavily muscled arms more quickly in an unpracticed movement than could a group of athletic physical education students, and that both the weight lifters and the physical education students moved more quickly than a group of relatively muscleless liberal arts students. As to the danger of weight lifting, Dr. Karpovich found in a survey of 31,702 lifters that most injuries were minor, consisting of "pulled" muscles and tendons. No heart injury was found in the survey, and the incidence of hernias among the lifters was twenty times less than would have been expected among an average group of people.

It should be noted, however, that no exercise or athletic activity can be completely risk free. Just as one can slip and be killed by a fall in the bathtub, one can be injured in any vigorous activity. The more vigorous the activity and the greater the participant's ambition, the greater the risk. A competing weight lifter risks injury for the possible glory of winning, just as any other athlete does.

A number of studies have shown that training exclusively for strength does not have as much cardiovascular effect as training exclusively by jogging. This fact is not surprising, and it is part of the basis for my recommendation that some jogging or rope skipping or cycling be incorporated in a training program to improve general physical fitness. No one has determined conclusively, however, that the physiological changes produced by one of these two types of training can be equated with what one might call "good health" to any greater extent than the changes produced by the other, or that one type of training will cause a person to live longer than another. If it should prove necessary to push a stalled automobile or move a heavy piece of furniture, I would hope that the person called upon for the effort will have put in as much time exercising with weights as he has with jogging.

Weight training does have a measurable effect on body function (other than strength) that other types of exercise have not been shown to have. Dr. Fred Abbo found that weight training maintains the ratio of certain hormones at a "youthful" level. Dr. Abbo first determined, in a study of a large group of men between the ages of twenty and eighty, that the ratio of 17-ketosteroids (17-KS) to 17-hydroxycorticosteroids (17-OHCS) tends to decline as men grow older. In subsequent studies, he found that this decline in natural hormone production may be preventable or postponable by training with weights. He found that such endurance exercises as handball, calisthenics, running, and swimming did not prevent the decline, but that exercising with weights three times a week did prevent it. Dr. Abbo also studied the effects of different kinds of exercise on a single subject, a forty-year-old man whose progress was followed for more than a year. The man did calisthenics and ran one or two miles three to five times a week for a year without achieving the "youthful" steroid level. Then weight training was added to his training, and the ratio established as normal for young men was attained within four months.

As Dr. Abbo concluded, his results did not definitely establish a special value for weight training, but they did suggest that this type of exercise does more than merely build muscles. Regular practitioners of weight training have believed this for decades, but no scientific studies have been conducted to determine effects on "health" as opposed to effects on muscular strength and size.

WHAT HAPPENS WHEN YOU STOP?

For some reason, people who know nothing about weight training generally seem to think that some terrible fate awaits the man who lifts weights for a time and then stops. Doesn't all that muscle turn to fat? is one question that is asked. The answer is that it does not. Muscle is muscle, and fat is fat. A person who does not exercise, or who exercises and then stops, tends to lose muscle size and strength. And a person who takes in more calories than he or she expends in activity takes on fat. But this has nothing specifically to do with weight lifting. The amount of fat and the shape of the body depend to a great extent on somatotype. The shape can be modified by exercise, but if you stop, your body tends to return to the shape it would have been in if you had never exercised. Former football players who stop exercising and eat too much get fat. So do former runners and tennis players, though if they are predominantly ectomorphic they remain more slender than larger-framed people. The fact that you have exercised has nothing to do with what happens when you don't exercise. Some of the fattest people of all have never lifted weights or participated in any other strenuous sport.

What happens when you don't stop? is the more interesting question, since most of the value of any exercise—the conditioning effect—is lost after the exerciser becomes inactive. I believe strength gained from weight training may last longer than endurance gained from running, but this is just an empirical observation since I don't know of any definitive scientific studies comparing the ef-

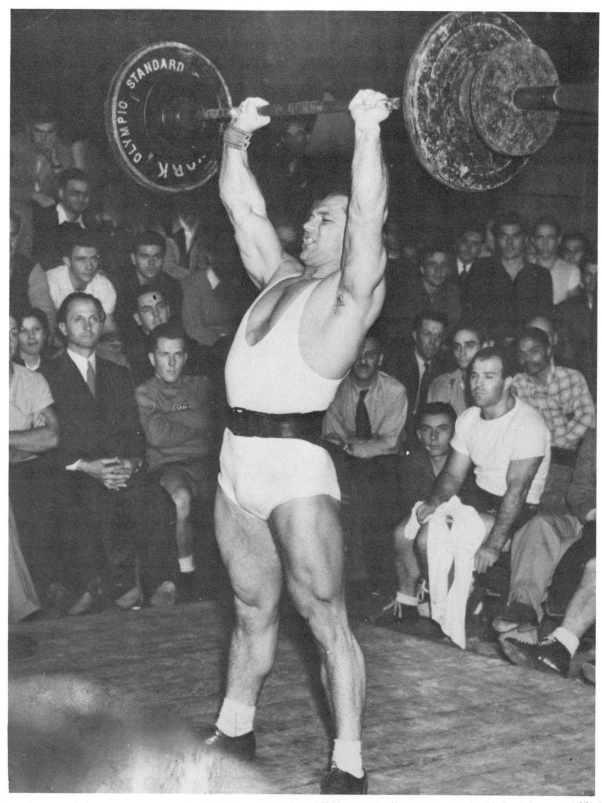

Fig. 6. This photo showing John Grimek pressing a heavy barbell was taken in 1940 when he was thirty years old—almost thirty years before the unposed snapshot that shows him as he looked in 1967. Grimek was a national weight lifting champion, a member of the 1936 Olympic team, and an undefeated winner of all major best-built-man contests.

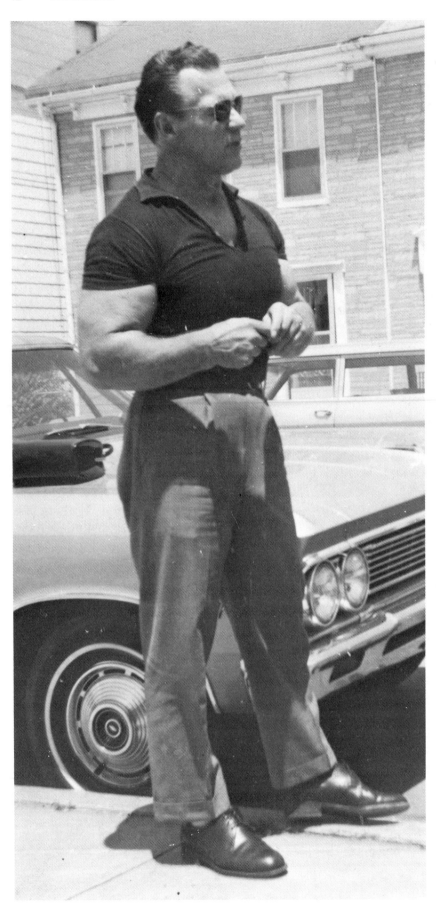

Fig. 7. This snapshot of John Grimek at 57 shows his ageless muscles. He retained the same massive chest and arms and exceptionally trim waist at 65!

fects of layoffs from different types of training. What we do know, from observation of individuals who continue weight training, is that such exercise is an excellent way to maintain above-average strength and a more youthful appearance for many, many years.

An outstanding example of this was provided by the experience of John Grimek, who was a national weight lifting champion and a member of the 1936 Olympic weight lifting team, and who later held the Mr. America and Mr. Universe titles. Grimek won Mr. America titles at thirty and thirty-one and the Mr. Universe crown at thirty-eight, ages when most men allow themselves to be "over the hill" physically. In his late thirties, Grimek defeated other Mr. America winners a decade younger, including such outstanding competitors as the superbly built Steve Reeves, who later won fame as a motion picture Hercules. Although his occupation as an editor of *Strength & Health* and *Muscular Development* magazines was sedentary, John Grimek was far from the typical out-of-shape type usually found in such white-collar occupations. In his forties, he moderated his training from exercise with 300-pound barbells for his arms and 400- to 500-pound barbells for his legs to work mostly with what were, to him, "light" weights. "Light" is relative, however, and I often marveled at the ease with which he did high repetition presses with a pair of 75-, 90-, or 100-pound dumbbells while lying against an inclined exercise bench.

The point is, continuing his exercise program seemed to have the effect of suspending John Grimek in time. After not seeing him for some years, I dropped in to visit John and found him apparently unchanged—still working to meet his magazine deadlines, still exercising "moderately," and still looking like a healthy man of forty-five with the body of a well-trained thirty-year-old. His chest was deep, his waist trim and muscular, his arms massive and powerful looking. But John Grimek was sixty-five!

The Grimek example is exceptional, but not isolated. Other men who have continued exercise have maintained great vitality for many years. Siegmund Klein, a famous strongman of the post-World War I era, maintained a fine gymnasium in New York City until he was seventy. After he "retired," he continued to work part-time as an instructor at another gymnasium. Arnold Schwarzenegger, who gained fame as a Mr. Universe and Mr. Olympia winner and as star of the movie *Pumping Iron,* worked out with Sig Klein and reported that Klein went through an entire body building routine with him—using lighter weights of course. Klein weighed about 150 pounds, Schwarzenegger more than 200. Klein was in his mid-seventies, Schwarzenegger in his late twenties!

Another old-timer who refused to surrender to Father Time was Karl Norberg. A longshoreman of great natural strength, Norberg dabbled in weight lifting for years, but practiced it most regularly after he retired from his strenuous occupation. Norberg suffered leg injuries in his work that made it impossible for him to jog or perform any of the kinds of exercise generally considered necessary for long-term "health." Instead, he lifted heavy weights, usually in a seated position or while lying supine. In his early seventies, Norberg could bench press more than 400 pounds. In his early eighties, he could still bench press more than 300 pounds! These are feats beyond the reach of most men at any age, but they do indicate that strength can be maintained much longer than most people have believed possible.

Do you suppose people ever asked Karl Norberg if he wasn't aware of the terrible life-shortening effects of his weight-lifting activities?

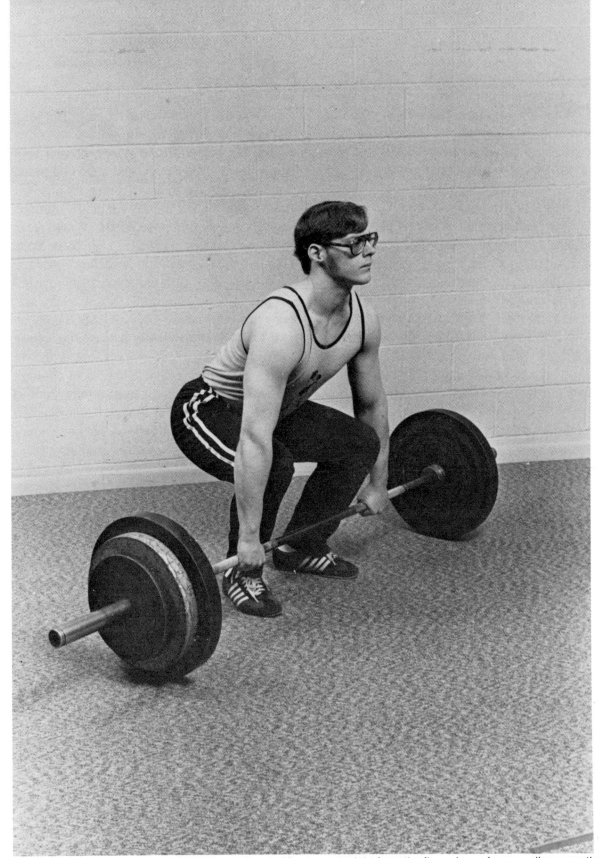

Fig. 8. Jay Murray shows perfect starting position to lift a heavy weight from the floor. Jay, a former college wrestler, demonstrated the power clean with 250 pounds for the photos, but has done 300—100 pounds more than his weight.

chapter 2
BASIC WEIGHT TRAINING

Certain basic weight training exercises are essential to build a foundation before beginning competitive weight lifting. The same exercises are important for building the balanced strength needed in any vigorous sport. And the same basic program also develops strength needed for total physical fitness and tones all the muscles of the body in such a way that the shape—the appearance—of both men and women improves.

There are many excellent pieces of equipment that have been designed to simulate weight training with a barbell. Some of them make certain exercises easier or more comfortable to perform; some provide resistance at a variety of angles, so that the muscles work harder over all or part of the range of motion; and all confine and restrict the random motion of the resistance so that they tend to be safer than working with a barbell. When special pieces of apparatus are available, as in gymnasiums and health clubs, it makes sense to take advantage of their convenience. It is important to realize, however, that none of them can provide all the power-building benefit of a free-moving barbell, which permits full neuromuscular expression of the exerciser's capacities. Lifting a barbell in any of the endless varieties of ways in which weights can be lifted incorporates acceleration and requires control, both essential elements in competitive weight lifting and other athletic sports.

CORRECT LIFTING POSITION AND THE POWER CLEAN

Pulling a barbell from the floor to the chest is the simplest description of a power clean. Correct performance of this exercise is important for a number of reasons. It teaches lifting technique for raising any heavy object; it is a key movement in training for athletic events that require great total body and leg power; and it incorporates the fundamental move of competitive weight lifting.

In essence, you perform a power clean by standing close to a barbell, crouching and grasping the bar with an even, comfortable

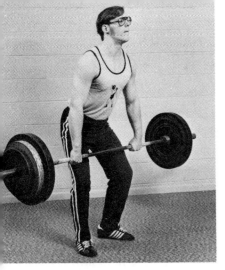

Fig. 9. This is the start of the "second pull" described in the text, the point at which the barbell is accelerated upward in the power clean.

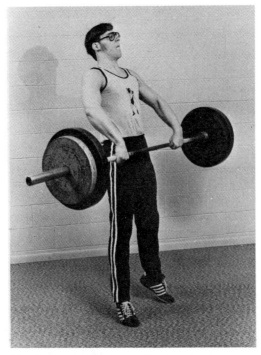

Fig. 10. A complete leg and back extension—including a quick rise-on-toes—powers the barbell upward. This photo shows a warm-up lift with 205 pounds. It is included in the series to show the full extension as the arms finish the pull.

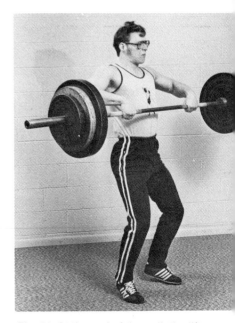

Fig. 11. At the end of the pull, the lifter bends his knees to cushion the shock when the weight strikes his chest. Note that the arms are just starting to turn the barbell over.

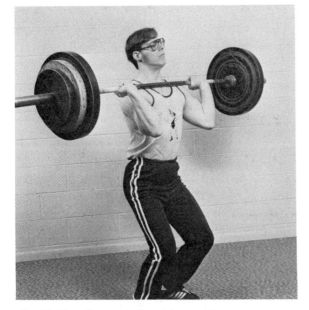

Fig. 12. The elbows are thrust forward to secure the lift as the barbell strikes the lifter's chest. Note the approximately one-quarter bend of the legs to help catch the weight smoothly.

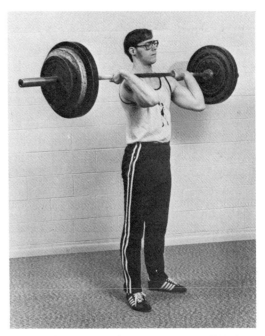

Fig. 13. Completion of the power clean. This is a great total-body exercise. It especially develops the back and legs for athletic moves requiring great body power and quick extension.

hand spacing, and then pulling it up to your chest. That is the essence, but the lift is actually much more complex, and each of its component parts is worthy of careful attention.

First, the starting position. Stand close to the barbell, so close that you can see the toes of your shoes extending past the bar as you look down. Your feet should be a comfortable distance apart, pointing straight ahead or toeing out slightly. The best distance apart is about the width of your hips. Bend forward and grasp the bar with an overhand grip, knuckles away from you. Your hands should be spaced so that, when the barbell is at your chest, your hands will be just outside your shoulders, not resting on them. You will have to experiment to find the exact hand spacing and foot spacing that is best for you. Some people feel more comfortable and function more efficiently when their feet are closer together than hip width; some function better with a slightly wider foot spacing. Exact hand spacing must also be determined by individual preference.

Closeness to the bar also varies slightly from one individual to another. Some pull best from a starting position in which their shins actually brush the bar when they get set to pull with their legs bent. Others function better a bit farther back, so that they do not quite touch the bar when they are set to lift.

Once the feet and hands are placed, body and leg position is extremely important. At the start of the pull from the floor, two features are essential: (1) the hip joints should be lower than the shoulder joints and (2) the back, especially the lower back (lumbar area) should be flat. People of different sizes and limb-to-trunk ratios may look quite different while meeting these two essentials. A tall, long-legged person will not be able to achieve as erect a body position as a shorter person whose trunk is long in relation to his arms and legs. The angle at which the back is inclined is not as important as meeting the two essentials—hips lower than shoulders and back flat.

From the starting position, you begin to lift by extending (straightening) your legs and back—with your back remaining flat throughout. Your arms should not jerk at the resting barbell, but should remain hanging loosely straight, hands gripping the bar firmly, as the barbell is started upward with the impetus of your leg and back extension.

As the barbell reaches knee height, you should consciously begin to pull with your arms, keeping the bar close to your thighs and body as it comes up. While pulling with your arms as the weight passes your thighs and body, you should try to accelerate the movement of the barbell. This effort becomes a total one as the weight passes in front of your body. At that point, you should have fully extended your legs and risen on your toes, and your hips should be thrust forward so that your back is actually hyperextended (arched slightly backward).

At the precise moment when the weight is as high as you can pull it with your arms bent and elbows high, legs and body extended, you should whip your elbows quickly down under the barbell, ramming them forward past it to turn the bar over and fix it securely at your chest. At the same time, you should dip at the knees to bring your hips back under the barbell and cushion the impact when it strikes your upper chest.

Many people, especially quick and well-coordinated athletes, will tend to jump slightly off the floor at the height of the pull. They may replace their feet exactly where they started from or jump them slightly sideways at the height of the pull. This is a natural reaction by a well-coordinated individual. If the leg dip under the barbell becomes more than a quarter bend, the exerciser needs to pay more attention to pulling and may in fact be trying to use too much weight. A deeper squat to receive the weight at the chest in the clean is a competitive weight lifter's technique and will be discussed later.

After the weight is cleaned, drop it from your chest to your thighs, controlling the drop with your arms and bending your legs so that it does not strike your thighs with a hard impact. Then lower it to the floor (if you are doing only one clean or intend to do repetitions from the floor) or to just above or below the knees for repetitions from that position. In lowering the weight, you should maintain the same flat-back position as when pulling it upward.

The complexities of this simple-appearing lift are well worth learning, for this is one of the very best power-building exercises, it is an essential preliminary to lifting a barbell overhead, and the basic elements apply to lifting anything heavy, such as a piece of furniture, a packing case, or machinery. The basics again: Keep a flat back with your hips lower than your shoulders; don't yank the barbell off the floor; start with a leg and back extension, then accelerate and follow through with your arms to finish the clean to the chest. It is so important to keep a flat back that you should try to actually arch it inward like a bow, forcing your chest and abdomen to protrude slightly. Unless you have a natural lordosis (inward curve of the low back), which is an asset to competitive weight lifters, you won't be able to arch your back inward very much. But by trying to do so, you will achieve the flat-back position you need for most efficient lifting with minimal danger of straining your lower back.

How much weight should you use to learn the power clean? The exact amount varies from one person to another, but it should be a light weight for that individual. It should be light enough that you can go through the lift smoothly, in "slow motion," yet heavy enough to give you a sensation of lifting. The competitive lifter can learn technique with a broomstick, but this is different: you need to feel some resistance in order to learn the motion properly. A bar with a 10-pound plate on either end—weighing a total of 25 to 65 pounds, depending on the type of bar—is probably enough to start with. Small plates make the starting position difficult because you have to bend low to reach the bar; so you will find yourself more comfortable in the starting position when you can handle 25-pound or heavier plates on the bar. Two 25-pound plates and a typical exercise bar have a total weight of 65 to 70 pounds. The same weights and an Olympic bar (which weighs 45 pounds) total 95 pounds.

Cleans should be done for three to five repetitions, emphasizing correct position and performance throughout. Once you have learned the technique, you should increase the weight by 10 pounds at a time (5 pounds on each end of the bar), continuing to do three repetitions with each weight until you feel that you cannot complete three correctly.

A typical series of weights and repetitions —called sets—for a beginner might be as follows: 65 pounds/five repetitions, 75/three, 85/three, 95/two, 100/one plus one (two single lifts). A more advanced weight trainer, perhaps a strong football player or wrestler on an off-season conditioning program, might do the following on an Olympic barbell: 135/ five, 155/five, 165/three, 175/three, 185/ two, 195/one, 200/one. This latter routine could only be followed by an exceptionally strong and well-conditioned athlete, and a fairly large one to boot. A reasonably strong person merely seeking to keep in condition with a 100-pound barbell could do so by lifting 70 to 80 pounds for five repetitions to warm up and then using the full 100 pounds for three to five sets of five or a single set of eight to ten repetitions.

Five to ten repetition cleans with 100 pounds represents fairly good strength. Five with 150 to 200 pounds represents enough strength to perform effectively on most high school or college athletic teams. A good goal for a healthy young athlete is to perform a single power clean with a barbell equal to his own weight. This will be harder for large people than for small ones, but it is within the reach of athletic and healthy young men of any size. A more ambitious goal is to clean 20 to 50 pounds more than body weight, and this is the kind of strength possessed by superior athletes. For example, one quick, well-coordinated eighteen year old weighing 240 pounds could power clean 280 pounds and put the high school shot more than 64 feet. This athlete, Dick Hart, also signed a bonus contract to play baseball with the Braves and later was a starting offensive lineman with the Philadelphia Eagles (where he made the national All-Rookie team as a guard his first year) and the Buffalo Bills. When Dick was playing professional football at 250 pounds, he could clean 310 pounds. After he retired from football, he continued exercising to keep in shape and progressed to clean 335. I mention this example to place in perspective the kind of athletic accomplishment associated with the ability to power clean 40 to 60 pounds more than body weight.

Even if you set a goal of using no more than 100 pounds in the power clean, you should work toward it gradually and progressively. For example, if you begin with the 65-75-85-95-100 pound series listed above, doing 5-3-3-2-1-1 repetitions and single lifts, you should stay with the same weights and attempt to add repetitions. Increase repetitions to 5-4-3-3-2 and 5-5-4-3-2 and 5-5-5-3-3, and so on until you can do five on the last set with 100 pounds. By then, you should be able to warm up with 70 to 80 pounds and do four or five more sets of as many repetitions as possible, to a maximum of five, with 100 pounds.

If you are working with heavier poundages and are ambitious to work up to the absolute limit of your potential, the approach must be more varied and must take into account your body's need for progressing in cycles. You should occasionally drop back to easier workouts to allow your body to recuperate and establish favorable neuromuscular patterns before moving on to heavier weights.

For example, if you use the advanced series listed above, working with 135 to 200 pounds in a series of five-five-three-three-two-one-one repetitions and single cleans, the set in which additional repetitions should be tried is the fifth, with 185 pounds. After

you move up from two to three repetitions in this set, it should be possible to get two with 195 on the sixth set in a subsequent workout. When you can do two with 195, it is time to try for a single lift with 205 on the final set. The sets then would be 135/five, 155/five, 165/three, 175/three, 185/three, 195/two, 205/one.

Dropping Back as Part of the Cycle

After having improved significantly in the amount of weight you can handle in the power clean or another exercise, it is a good idea to take one or two lighter workouts before starting to work up again from the new peak performance. For example, if you reach the peak performance described in the last paragraph, you might drop back to 135/five, 150/five, 160/three, and three sets of three repetitions with 170 pounds. Then move up slightly, to 135/five, 155/three, 165/three, 175/two, and three single cleans with 190. Next, repeat the peak workout, but increase the weight five pounds on the fifth and sixth sets, trying for 135/five, 155/five, 165/three, 175/three, 190/two, 200/one, and attempting 210. Work at this sequence until you can increase the repetitions to three with 190 pounds and two with 200. When you can do 190/three, 200/two, and 210/one on the final sets, it is time to drop back for two easy workouts and then work to surpass your previous peak, adding five pounds to every set except the first. One hundred thirty-five pounds (an Olympic bar and two 45-pound plates) is plenty for anyone to warm up with. Many world champion weight lifters begin warming up with an unloaded bar, 45 pounds, and then proceed to 65 and 95 pounds before placing the big 45-pound plates on the bar. These are men whose workouts include snatches with 300 pounds or more and cleans with more than 400 pounds.

Space limitation makes it impossible to describe cyclic progression in any more detail. Besides, any progression program must be individualized. The essential points to keep in mind are these: Work in sets of five, three, two, and single lifts unless you intend to keep the weight moderate, for conditioning only. As a conditioning exercise, cleans can be done five to ten repetitions. The total number of cleans should be in the range of 15 to 30, whether they are done in sets of five, using light weights, or working with decreasing repetitions, using heavier weights. With the heavier weights, try to coax your body along to greater power by increasing the repetitions from two to three and from one to two. After successfully adding repetitions on the final sets, you are ready to try for a new personal record. After achieving it, or anytime you feel sluggish or stale during a workout, decrease the weight a few pounds and take one or two workouts. Then revise the entire series upward and begin the progression again.

Obviously, no progression can continue indefinitely. Eventually you will reach a level that you cannot exceed except for occasional small improvements on especially good days. At this point, you should cycle your workouts weekly. Schedule a light day for using weights 60 to 70 percent as heavy as those used on your best days, a moderate day for weights that are 70 to 80 percent of your best, and a heavy day for working with resistance weighing 90 to 105 percent of your best.

AN ALTERNATE APPROACH: THE DEAD LIFT

If you find the power clean too difficult to learn or too strenuous, you can perform a simple exercise with an ominous name, the dead lift, as an alternative. To do this exercise, assume the same starting position as for the clean and raise the weight smoothly, without acceleration, only to the height of your thighs as you stand erect with your shoulders back. Very heavy weights can be lifted in this exercise, especially if you turn one hand around, palm away from you, and keep the other in an overhand grip. This hand placement will assist your grip and permit repetitions that might otherwise be difficult because you were having trouble holding on to the barbell. If you proceed cautiously, you can do this exercise in ''poor form''—that is, with your hips high, back rounded, and knees only slightly bent, to deliberately (and carefully!) stretch the muscles of your lower back and the hamstrings at the backs of your thighs.

I do not recommend that you lift heavy weights in the dead lift—even though heavy-weight lifters have raised 700 to 800 pounds and more—because I believe such weights put too much strain on the lower back. But three sets of five to ten repetitions with 100 pounds should be safe for anyone with no structural inadequacies, and sets of three to five with 200 to as much as 400 pounds are probably safe for strong athletes who maintain a flat back and keep their hips low while lifting. The problem with heavy dead lifts is that you cannot keep your back flat when lifting weights at your limit, and there is always the temptation to see how much you can do. A painful lumbosacral strain is more likely to result from such exercise than from heavy cleans. However, the quick movement in the clean does expose you to some risk of muscle or ligament strain.

OVERHEAD PRESS, FOR SHOULDER POWER

We devoted many pages to the power clean because it is a very important lift and should be done properly for best results and to minimize the likelihood of strains and ''pulls''— the minor muscle injuries that are so annoying, mainly because they impede progress. The clean is also important because it is used to get the weight to the shoulders for the next basic exercise: the overhead press. Pressing overhead used to be more popular than it is today, before it was eliminated as a part of weight lifting competition and before special benches became available to make supine pressing more convenient. The overhead

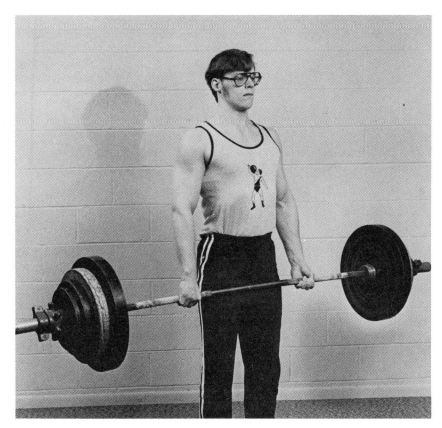

Fig. 14. This photo shows the completion of the dead lift, which begins with the same starting position as shown for the power clean. In the dead lift, however, the hands may be alternated (one overhand and one underhand) for a more secure grip.

press is still an important exercise, however, because it is highly effective in developing the deltoid muscles that cap the shoulders, especially the front part of the deltoids.

The press is much easier to learn than the clean. First clean the weight to your chest, hands a bit wider apart than shoulder width. Then thrust your hips forward slightly, tensing your buttocks, low back, and thighs, and push the barbell smoothly overhead. Keep it as close to your face as possible, and shift your body forward slightly as the barbell passes the top of your head, so that you finish standing erect with your arms straight up under the weight.

Begin with eight repetitions and work up to twelve by adding a repetition during every workout that you feel able to do so. When you can do twelve, add five or ten pounds—whichever limits you to eight repetitions—and begin the progression again.

As you begin to make progress after three to six workouts, your muscles will need more work than they get from one set. Add a second set of eight to ten repetitions with the same weight, or add five or ten pounds to the barbell for a second set of six to eight repetitions. As two sets become easy, add a third. If you use the same weight for all three sets, the third set should consist of eight to ten repetitions. If you add five to ten pounds for each set, you will probably not be able to do more than three to six repetitions for the third set.

To obtain the best bodybuilding effect with presses, do three sets of eight to twelve repetitions. To emphasize strength and power, add weight for each set and decrease the repetitions. If you use weights heavy enough to limit the repetitions to five or less, add enough sets to bring the total number of presses to at least twenty.

Although it is very satisfying to press ever heavier weights, it is also important to keep the exercise a true press. That is, keep your legs locked in position and try to stand fairly

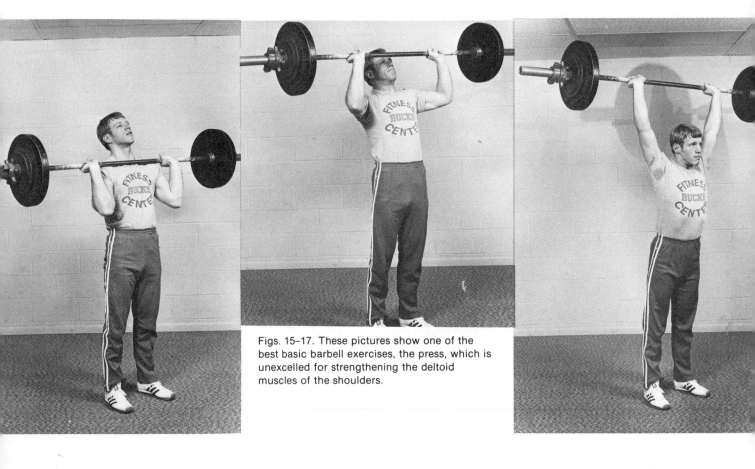

Figs. 15–17. These pictures show one of the best basic barbell exercises, the press, which is unexcelled for strengthening the deltoid muscles of the shoulders.

straight while you press, even though you can lift more by "kicking" (quickly unlocking and straightening your legs) and by bending away from the weight as it goes up. The more you loosen up in performance, by kicking, bending, or both, the more the exercise affects your whole body and the less direct benefit there is to the shoulders. There is no need to press deliberately slowly, but you should try to do all the work with your shoulders and arms. For variety, you can take a slightly wider grip and begin the press with the weight in back of your shoulders, lifting it behind your head.

How much weight should you be able to press? A press with seventy-five percent of your own body weight is very good, and a press with ninety percent of your weight is excellent, especially for people of heavier body weight. Ninety percent would be 135 pounds for a person weighing 150 and 180 pounds for a 200-pounder. A goal of press-

ing a barbell equal to body weight is within reach for people with favorable leverage, and champion weight lifters have lifted 100 to 200 pounds more than their weight in presses of various degrees of strictness. Paul Anderson, the great strongman and Olympic champion from Georgia, who usually weighed from 300 to 350 pounds, could perform very strict presses with more than 400 pounds and could lift 500 or more with a jerk-press that included only a slight knee kick to start the weight moving. For a person who is not a weight lifting specialist, however, pressing from 10 to 50 pounds more than body weight is a very impressive feat. A press of 50 pounds more than body weight certainly represents enough strength for a well-coordinated and motivated athlete to succeed in any sport, including sports requiring great power, such as shot-putting.

For general fitness, ten presses with 100 pounds is a good maintenance level to strive for. The ability to press 150 pounds ten times represents superior strength, certainly enough for a college athlete, even in football and wrestling, except in the most highly competitive conferences.

THE PARALLEL SQUAT, FOR UNPARALLELED POWER

Squatting—performing knee bends with a barbell held low behind your neck across the shoulders—is not much fun, but it is the key exercise for developing great leg strength and power. There has been some controversy about this exercise because certain exercise physiologists believe deep squats—all the way down—overstretch the knees' supporting structures and make them more vulnerable to injuries. This controversy is not satisfactorily resolved, but it doesn't matter. Those who have no need to go into a deep squat as a competing weight lifter does can derive great benefit by bending their knees only until their thighs are approximately parallel with the floor.

It should be noted that there is little evidence that deep squats themselves cause any damage to the knees. Champion lifters who drop into and rebound from full squats very quickly with heavy weights seem to have fewer knee problems than many other athletes, especially football players. It may be, however, that stretching the knees with deep squats makes a football player's knees somewhat looser and therefore more vulnerable to injury from quick changes of direction on cleated shoes or from blows against the sides of the legs. For this reason, athletes who are not seeking competitive weight lifting proficiency or the full thigh development needed in bodybuilding contests are advised to place a knee-high object behind them when they do squats and to begin to rise as soon as they feel the object. An exercise bench makes a good "stopper," as is shown in Fig. 18.

Performance of the squat exercise is as follows. Place a barbell on supports a bit lower

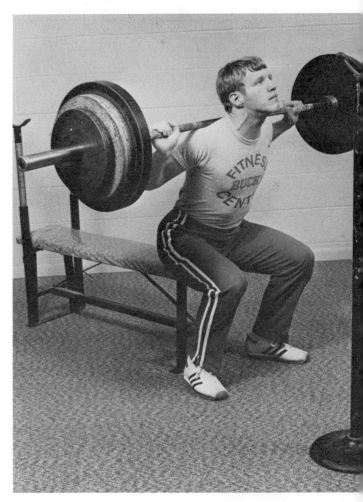

Fig. 18. Squatting to build leg strength is effective as long as the bend is approximately to a point where the thighs are parallel with the floor. Many coaches and trainers recommend the use of a knee-high bench to remind the exerciser not to go any lower.

than shoulder height and load it to the proper poundage. The weight should be enough to feel difficult after three or four repetitions, but not so heavy as to prevent you from completing at least eight. Place your hands evenly on the bar, farther apart than shoulder width, and duck under the bar so that your head is centered and the barbell rests across your shoulders, low at the back of the neck. It should be kept low so it doesn't rest perceptibly on a protruding vertebra, a position that can be uncomfortable at best. (Some people prefer to wrap the center of the bar with a towel for added comfort.)

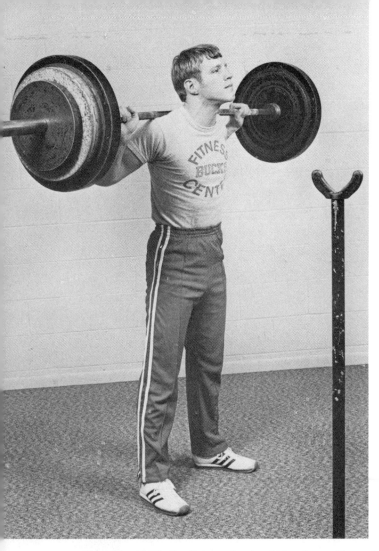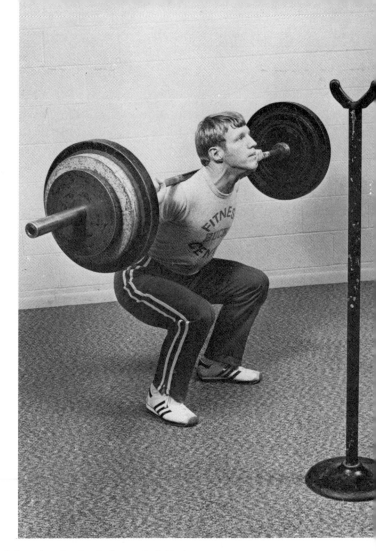

Figs. 19 and 20. Parallel squats should be done with control, keeping the back flat and sinking until the tops of the thighs are about horizontal, then rising.

With the bar solidly across the back of your shoulders, straighten your legs to clear the weight from the supports and step back one or two short steps, far enough so that when you squat down, leaning forward slightly, the bar doesn't contact the supports. Place your feet about hip-width apart and either pointing straight ahead or toeing out slightly. As in the clean, you will have to experiment to find the most comfortable and efficient foot position. Then take a breath high in the chest, trying to hold your waist in and keeping your back arched slightly or flat, but never rounded. Squat so that the tops of your thighs are approximately parallel to the floor. Then rise immediately. Begin to exhale after you start to push upward. When your

legs are straight, pause, breathe deeply (but high in your chest) again, and repeat the desired number of times. You should try to work up from eight to twelve or fifteen repetitions. Then add weight, drop back to eight, and repeat the progression.

If you do squats when you are alone, be sure you can complete the repetitions you are attempting. It is preferable to have one or two ''spotters'' to help you get up if you should lose balance or be unable to rise with a heavy weight.

The amount of weight used differs greatly from one individual to another. As a general conditioning exercise for your legs, you might do the parallel squat with a 100-pound barbell across your shoulders for one to three sets of from ten to fifteen repetitions (twenty if you're really ambitious). As with any exercise, a beginner will have to experiment with lighter weights to find the right poundage at which to begin progression in building strength. In addition to working up to three sets of eight to twelve or fifteen repetitions with progressively heavier weights, you can build great leg strength and power by working with no more than five repetitions per set · and striving to increase the poundage in cycles, as described for the power clean.

For example, a strong young athlete who can do three sets of ten repetition squats with 150 pounds might practice the following routine: 135 pounds/five repetitions to warm up, then 150/five, 165/five, 175/three, 190/two, and 200/one. In subsequent workouts, repetitions should be added, one or two at a time as you feel able, to the fourth, fifth, and final set. When you can do five repetitions in the first five sets and three with 200, adjust the entire series upward as follows: 135/five, 160/five, 180/five, 195/three, 205/two, and 210/one. Then try to add repetitions on the final three sets as before. During this kind of progression, you should occasionally take one or two easier workouts, especially after establishing a new peak performance. An easier workout might consist of 135/eight, 155/eight, 175/six to eight, and 190/three.

You have to learn to feel your way along as you progress in building strength, and only experience can tell you when to ease off and when to move ahead. You have to learn the difference between cutting back because you are lazy and cutting back to avoid staleness. The former should be avoided, but the latter is absolutely necessary, and nothing is more self-defeating than to try to force yourself to progress simply because you have planned to do so on a given day. A good instructor or perceptive training partner can help with making such judgments, for it is often very difficult to persuade yourself that an easier workout would be beneficial during an upward cycle when you are feeling strong.

What are the ultimate possibilities in the squat? The poundages that have been lifted in this exercise are mind-bending. As an example of absolute strength, consider the 1,200 pounds that massive Paul Anderson squatted with a few years ago. Anderson, of course, had a leverage and structure that ideally suited him for this exercise. At his height of approximately 5′ 10″ he weighed, usually, between 300 and 350 pounds— sometimes more! When he was twenty-one, Anderson had 9-inch wrists, 11½-inch ankles, and 21-inch knees. His powerful thighs, measuring 34 inches at the time, packed more muscle than most men could ever hope to acquire.

Another gigantic strongman, Vasily Alexeyev of Russia, was reported to have squatted with 1,014 pounds, and other superheavyweight lifters in power lifting competition, such as Don Reinhoudt, John Kuc, and Jon Cole, handled weights of from 800 to 900 pounds. People of more normal size (but with much more muscle than average people of the same weight) have also squatted with mind-boggling poundages. David Rigert, the Russian 198-pound world champion, was said to have squatted three repetitions with 672 pounds. Larry Pacifico, world power lifting champion in the 198 pound class, could do even more! Power lifting champions weighing 114 and 123 pounds have squatted with more than 400 pounds, and middleweights of 165 pounds (the best in the world, of course) have done squats with weights in the 500 to 600 pound range.

For more nearly average people, a squat with 20 to 50 pounds more than body weight is a commendable effort. But high-level athletic performance in sports demanding strength requires squats with 100 to 200 pounds more than body weight. It is doubtful that any champion shot-putter or professional football lineman would be adequately prepared for his sport unless he could squat to parallel with at least 400 pounds.

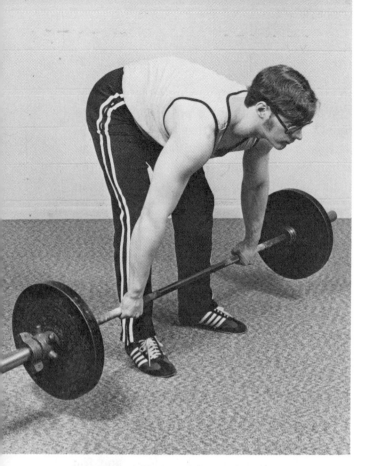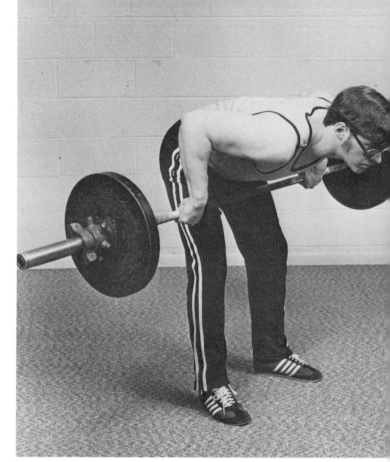

Figs. 21 and 22. the rowing motion strengthens the arms and the backs of the shoulders, but it is especially effective for developing the latissimus dorsi muscles, which add width to the back. The bar is pulled up to lightly touch at the upper abdomen.

ROWING, TO DEVELOP THE BACK MUSCLES

Oarsmen have always been noted for broad, well-muscled backs, and the best basic barbell exercise for the major upper back muscles is the rowing motion. This exercise is done while holding the barbell with an overhand grip and leaning forward from the hips so that the torso is parallel with the floor. Your hands should be spaced about shoulder-width apart, and you will be more comfortable if you bend your knees slightly to minimize strain on your lower back. You shouldn't bend your knees much, however, because when your arms are hanging down, the barbell should be just clear of the floor.

For the starting position, let the weight hang straight down under your chest. Then pull the barbell up and slightly toward your abdomen so that it touches below your chest but well up on your abdomen. You should feel your back muscles stretching as the weight goes down and contracting as you pull it up. It is important to consciously work your back muscles in this exercise; otherwise, it may be chiefly an arm exercise. No matter how effectively you perform the rowing motion, your arms will tire before your back does, even though the exercise is primarily intended to develop the big latissimus dorsi muscles that extend from under your arms well down along your sides to the lower back. These muscles pull your arms down and back and are also worked strongly by chinning and by the "latissimus machine" pulleys in gymnasiums. Rowing with a barbell is an especially good exercise, however, because it also develops allied back muscles between the latissimus dorsi muscles.

Learn the rowing motion with a weight

that you can handle fairly easily for eight repetitions. For most people, 35 to 50 pounds is enough to start with. Next, experiment to find a weight that is more demanding for eight repetitions, and then try to add repetitions with each workout until you reach twelve. When you can do twelve, add enough weight—probably 10 pounds—to restrict you to eight, and then work up to twelve again. In addition to increasing the number of repetitions, you should add sets, to three, after the workouts become easy.

For general fitness, 100 pounds is plenty of weight to use in the rowing exercise, even for a person who is stronger than average. The ability to do this exercise with from 120 to 150 pounds for 10 repetitions represents superior strength, but an aspiring weight lifter or wrestler may want to work up to a barbell equal to body weight or more. This is an especially good exercise for wrestlers, since the pull-in motion develops the strength needed to pull in a leg or arm in take-down or riding situations.

THE BENCH PRESS, KEY TO UPPER BODY STRENGTH

The supine press on bench is probably most weight trainers' favorite exercise. The main reasons for this are that it is especially effective for building strength and muscle size in the shoulders, chest, and arms; it enables the exerciser to work with poundages that are very satisfying to the ego; and, in addition, it can be done while lying down!

To do the exercise, you need a barbell and a sturdy bench, preferably one with uprights to hold the barbell, as shown in Figs. 23 and 24. If you have a bench without uprights, you'll need one or two strong training partners to hand you the barbell. Whether you have a bench with uprights or not, however, you should not try weights you are not absolutely certain you can lift unless you have someone standing by as a "spotter" to help you if you can't complete a press. This is

one of the more potentially dangerous exercises, since there is the temptation to try a few more pounds or one more repetition when no "spotter" is present. In rare instances, people have been killed after succumbing to this temptation, for if fatigued muscles fail, the bar can come to rest across the lifter's throat!

Aside from this hazard, which should not trouble a prudent person who knows his limitations, the bench press is a great exercise. You need a slightly wider grip in this exercise than in the standing press, but the grip shouldn't be excessively wide. It should place your forearms in a vertical position during the middle range of the press.

Start this exercise in the finishing position, taking the weight off the supports (or from training partners) and holding it briefly on straight arms that point directly up from your shoulders. Next, take a deep breath and lower the weight to touch the lower chest muscles, near where the pectoral muscles meet the abdomen. Then immediately push the weight back up so that your arms are straight. Begin to exhale as the weight goes up and take a breath while your arms are straight. Lower the weight to your chest and continue for eight to twelve repetitions. Experiment to find the correct starting weight for eight repetitions, beginning with a conservative poundage of about 35 to 50 pounds.

As you feel stronger, add repetitions to twelve and then add enough weight—probably ten pounds—to make eight repetitions feel difficult again. Add sets, too, as your condition improves, until you are doing three sets of eight to twelve. Incidentally, men who enter bodybuilding competition may do many more sets and repetitions than advocated here, but bodybuilding is not the subject of this book. Body builders also employ many little techniques to increase muscle tension and enhance development—for example, they may not quite lock their arms at the top of the press or lock for only a split sec-

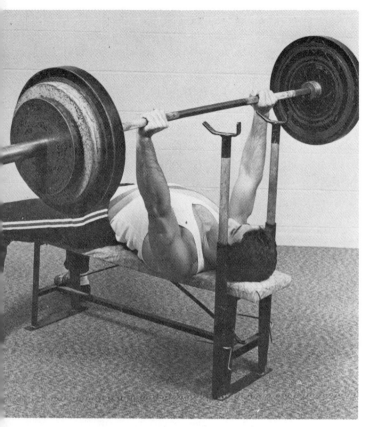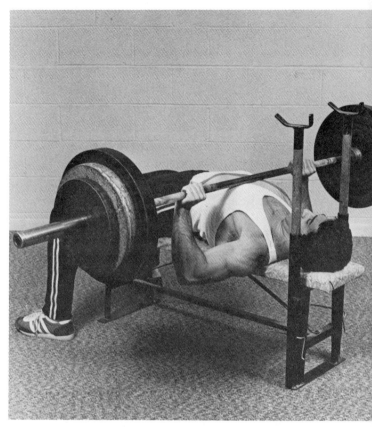

Figs. 23 and 24. The bench press is unexcelled for developing the muscles of the chest, shoulders, and arms. It begins with the barbell at straight arms. The bar is then lowered to touch the chest and pushed up to straight arms again.

ond—but this is not necessary for people seeking general fitness, strength, and power. A brief pause with fully locked arms allows you a moment to gather your resources for the next effort.

The bench press is another exercise in which a fitness seeker can be satisfied, and maintain a good strength level, with three sets of twelve repetitions with 100 pounds. Ten repetitions with 125 pounds is within many people's reach, however, and most athletic men can work up to a single bench press with a barbell equal to body weight or more. In fact, body weight plus 10 or 20 pounds is a good goal for a single press for athletic people of average structure. And 50 to 100 pounds more than body weight is well within the reach of athletes who have favorable pressing leverage. Some people who do

not look like "pressers" can handle surprising poundages in this exercise; Dave Wottle, who was an Olympic 800-meter running champion, bench pressed 180 pounds while weighing only 140. On the other hand, I knew a good college football player, a starting guard, who weighed 200 pounds and could bench press only about 10 pounds more than his own weight. However, even the person with poor leverage, who is handicapped in the amount of weight he can lift, derives great strength-building benefit from the exercise, and he can use the strength developed by weight training effectively in other ways.

The possibilities in the bench press, for strong, well-coordinated people with good leverage, are astounding. A number of college and professional football players have bench pressed 300, 400, or even 500 pounds.

Champion shot-putters and discus throwers also handle these kinds of weights. World class power lifters of 114 to 132 pounds bench press 220 to 300 pounds. The bigger men in the 181- and 198-pound classes bench press more than 400, and heavyweights and superheavies (over 242 pounds) bench press 500 or even 600 pounds!

If you want to work up to heavy poundages in the bench press, you must perform sets with increasing weights and decreasing repetitions as in the other lifts. For example, suppose you have progressed on a three-sets-of-eight-to-twelve system until you can do 150 pounds for ten repetitions, and you want to work up more quickly to heavier single lifts. You might try the following sequence: 120/eight, 135/five, 150/five, 160/three, 170/two or three, and 175/one or two. At each workout an effort should be made to increase the repetitions with 170 and 175 until you can comfortably do three bench presses with each weight. Then add a set, doing one press with 185 and striving for two whenever you feel able to do it. (Be sure to have one or two spotters on hand when you try limits.) When you can do two with 185, it is time to drop back for one or two easy workouts with, say, 120/eight, 140/eight, 160/two, 170/two plus two. Then adjust the whole series upward to 135/five, 150/five, 160/three to five, 175/two to five, and 190/one. When you can bench press 175/five and 190/two or three, drop back for a light workout and then move the series up again, except for the starting weight of 135/eight. That's enough to warm up with regardless of how much you eventually plan to work up to.

There are, incidentally, many combinations of sets and repetitions that you can use to make progress when you become stale on either three sets of eight to twelve or an 8-5-5-3-3-2-1 series. For specialized approaches to bodybuilding and power lifting (the bench press is a competition event in power lifting), read the books by Franco Columbu and Terry

Todd. Periodicals on weight training, power lifting, and weight lifting also provide different training approaches. Only by trying many different approaches can you continue to progress to ever higher accomplishments. However, the basic techniques described in this book provide the groundwork for bodybuilding, power competition, and Olympic weight lifting, which is covered later in the book. Periodicals that provide useful information on exercise and nutrition include the following:

Strength & Health
P.O. Box 1707
York, PA 17405

Muscular Development
P.O. Box 1707
York, PA 17405

Muscle Mag International
Unit One—270 Rutherford Rd.
Brampton, Ont., Canada

Iron Man
512 Black Hills Ave.
Alliance, NB 69301

Muscle Builder/Power
21100 Erwin St.
Woodland Hills, CA 91364

Muscle Training Illustrated
1665 Utica Ave.
Brooklyn, NY 11234

Coaching journals, such as *Scholastic Coach,* also include useful information on weight training, especially exercise programs for specialized athletic conditioning. Another source of information on weight training is *Track & Field News,* P.O. Box 296, Los Altos, CA 94022. Although this publication is devoted to track and field, so many runners, jumpers, and throwers become intensively involved in weight training that the magazine often describes lifting routines.

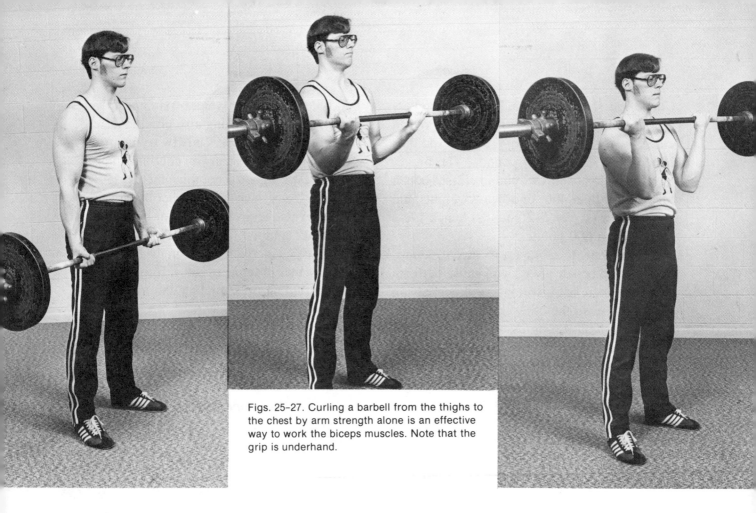

Figs. 25–27. Curling a barbell from the thighs to the chest by arm strength alone is an effective way to work the biceps muscles. Note that the grip is underhand.

THE CURL, FOR THE BICEPS AND FOREARMS

The biceps muscle, which lumps up when the arm is flexed in response to a request to ''show me your muscle,'' can be strengthened and increased in size by performing an exercise known as the curl. This exercise is done with palms away from the body, not with the overhand grip used for most lifting. After grasping the bar with an underhand grip, stand erect with your arms hanging straight and the bar across your thighs. Then flex your arms, keeping your elbows at your sides, so that the barbell moves in an arc from your thighs to your upper chest. Inhale before making the effort and begin exhaling as the bar passes through the middle of the range of motion, directly in front of your elbows.

Curls should be done with a weight that permits eight repetitions with difficulty. Add repetitions whenever you are able until you reach twelve, and then add five or ten pounds and begin again at eight repetitions. You should also add sets as you begin to make progress until you are doing three sets of eight to twelve.

Thirty to fifty pounds is enough for most people to start with in the curl, and seventy-five to eighty pounds for three sets of ten repetitions is enough to use for general conditioning. It takes a very strong person to curl 100 pounds ten repetitions, but much heavier weights are possible. Exceptionally strong bodybuilders and weight lifters have curled barbells loaded to as much as their own weight and a bit more. These were single curls, needless to say.

Certain variations of the curl are also useful, especially for developing the forearm muscles and strengthening the grip. One is to perform the exercise exactly as described except with an overhand grip. This variation is called the reverse curl. Most people can lift less with the reverse curl than with the curl, but during the 1940s a strongman named

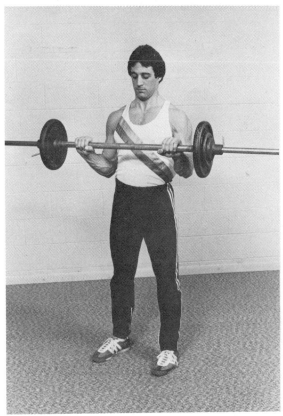

Fig. 28. When curls are done with an overhand grip—"reverse curls"—the exercise works the forearms strongly.

Al Berger, who was just under six feet tall and weighed about 200 pounds, succeeded in reverse curling a 177-pound barbell while standing strictly erect with legs straight and heels together in a position of attention. Berger had exceptionally strong hands and forearms and could chin himself by pinch gripping two-inch-thick boards!

Another variation is to sit with a light barbell in your hands, your forearms resting on your thighs and your hands extending past your knees. In this position, curl your wrists up and down as far as possible. Wrist curls involve the forearm muscles very strongly and should be done with both an underhand and an overhand grip. An unloaded bar is probably enough to start with in doing wrist curls, which should be done for ten to fifteen repetitions, two to three sets, with palms both up and down.

Curls can also be done very effectively with dumbbells. Start with the handles pointing fore and aft at the sides of your legs. Turn your palms up as you curl the weights upward, and finish with the dumbbells parallel with your collarbone and your palms in.

Fig. 29. This is the start of a wrist curl, in which a person develops his forearms by raising the barbell as far as possible with wrist motion only. Note that this picture shows an underhand grip, which allows a person to begin the lift with fingers extended.

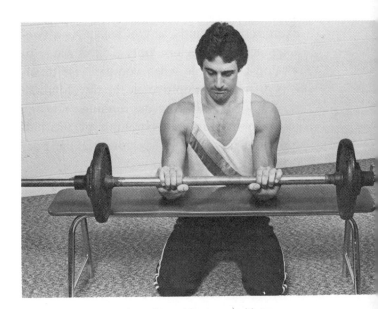

Fig. 30. The finish of a wrist curl is shown with an overhand grip. For a complete forearm workout, wrist curls should be done with both an overhand and an underhand grip.

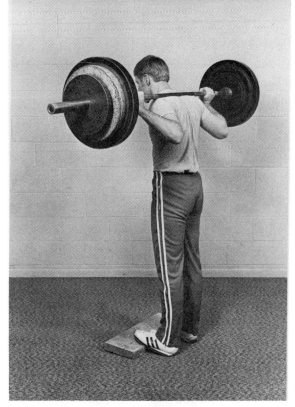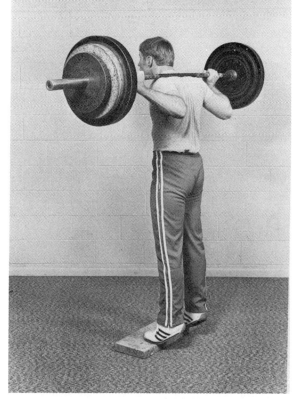

Figs. 31 and 32. These photos of the rise-on-toes exercise show the full range of motion that should be used to exercise the calf muscles and stretch the Achilles tendons. When this exercise is done with legs straight, the upper part of the calf (gastrocnemius) is worked strongly.

THE RISE-ON-TOES, FOR THE CALF MUSCLES

The muscles of the lower legs, the calves, are very dense and tough because they are exercised constantly as you walk. As a consequence, and because only a short range of motion is possible when you exercise them, it is difficult to improve on the development resulting from walking and running. You can increase the size and strength of the calf muscles, however, by performing the rise-on-toes exercise in two ways.

First, set a barbell across your shoulders as though you were going to do squats, and then place your toes and the balls of your feet on a thick board. Rise up on your toes and then let your heels down to touch the floor. Repeat from fifteen to twenty times. When this exercise is done with the legs straight, it develops the upper part of the calf muscle. When it is done with the legs bent, more work is done by the lower part of the muscle, near the Achilles tendon of the heel.

The second form of the rise-on-toes works the lower part of the calf very strongly. For this one, you must be seated, with a substantial pad on your thighs so you can place the barbell across them without hurting your legs. You again use a board under the front of the foot in order to obtain full stretch of the muscle as well as full contraction when you rise as high as possible on your toes.

Both standing and seated calf exercises should be done with as much weight as you can handle, and you should work up to three sets of fifteen to twenty repetitions. Best results are obtained with 150 to 250 pounds, but there is little value in using more weight than you can handle properly through a full range of motion. Fifty to 100 pounds is plenty of weight to start with.

In doing the rise-on-toes exercises, it is a good idea to change the position of your feet from set to set in order to activate the tough calf muscles fully. When you do the exercise with heels out and toes in, the outer parts of

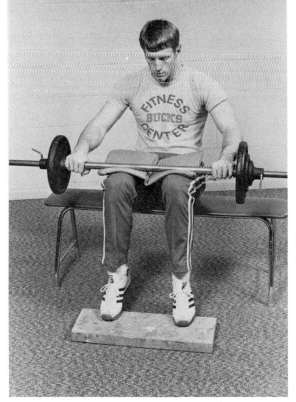

Fig. 33. To focus work on the lower portion of the calf muscle (soleus), the rise-on-toes exercise should be done as pictured, with the knees bent.

the muscles work harder. When you do it with heels in and toes out, the inner muscles work harder.

THE SIT-UP, FOR ABDOMINAL MUSCLES

In order to strengthen the muscles of your abdomen, you have to do an exercise that causes them to contract against resistance. However, the best exercise for this area— the sit-up—can be started without using weights because body leverage alone is enough for most people to overcome when they first start exercising.

To begin the exercise, lie supine with your feet anchored and your knees bent to approximately a right angle. The bent knees help flatten your lower back against the floor or sit-up board, which is where it should be as you start, and also relax muscles running from the thighs to the pelvis that would otherwise do a lot of the work and lessen the work of the abdominal muscles you are trying to strengthen.

Clasp your hands behind your head, inhale, and then exhale. As you exhale, pull your abdomen in, tilt your pelvis upward so your lower back presses against the floor or sit-up board, and "crunch" into a sit-up by bringing your head toward your chest and then rais-

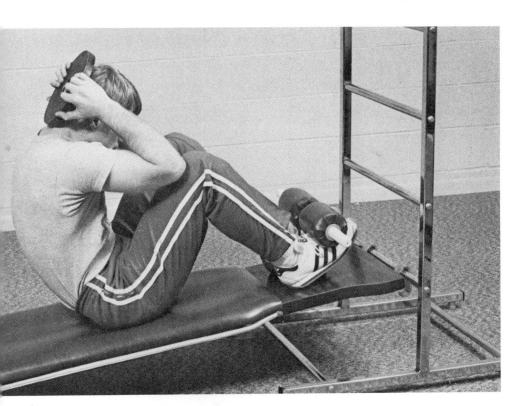

Fig. 34. Abdominal muscle strength is developed by sit-ups. Bending the knees inactivates muscles that help when the legs are kept straight. As a result, the abdomen does most of the work. The exercise is made more difficult by working "uphill" on a slant board and by holding a weight behind the head.

ing your upper back and curling up into a full sitting position, touching your elbows to your knees. Immediately uncurl, inhaling. Repeat 10 or 20 times. You can add to the effectiveness of the exercise by alternately touching your right elbow to your left knee and your left elbow to your right knee.

If you have trouble sitting up with your hands behind your head, reach forward with your hands; that will help you get up. If you can do only a few repetitions, say five, rest and repeat the exercise until you have done a total of 20 sit-ups.

If you can easily do 20 sit-ups with your hands behind your head, increase the repetitions to 25 the next time you exercise. Keep adding five until you can do 50 without stopping. Then do the exercise with a 5-pound weight behind your head, starting with 20 repetitions. Add repetitions until you can do 50 and then increase the weight until you are satisfied with the strength and firmness of your abdomen. Fifty sit-ups with a 10-pound weight behind the head is easily within most people's reach, if they work at the exercise. Many serious bodybuilders do hundreds of sit-ups, and a New York policeman named Frank Leight—who won a Mr. America title—once did a single sit-up (legs straight, feet held down) with 154 pounds held behind his head.

Incidentally, many authorities on physical training insist that abdominal exercises have no special merit for reducing fat on the abdomen. Theoretically they are correct, but in practice people can reduce their waistlines by performing sit-ups, because toning the abdominal muscles pulls them in so that they can keep the once-protruding abdomen under control. In addition, this exercise, like all exercise, helps to burn calories. The best way to reduce the abdomen, however, consists of a combination of cutting back caloric intake—especially of high-carbohydrate foods, continuous exercises that use up stored fat (jogging and steady walking are especially good), and exercises such as the sit-up that strengthen and pull in the sagging muscles.

THE PULL-OVER, FOR EXPANDING THE CHEST

A person can develop an impressive-looking chest by building the pectoral muscles that cover it. This can be done by bench presses

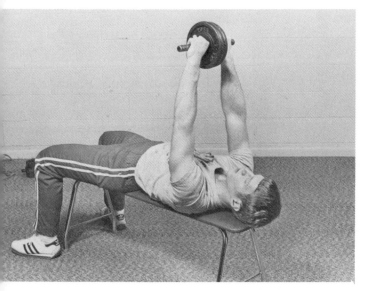
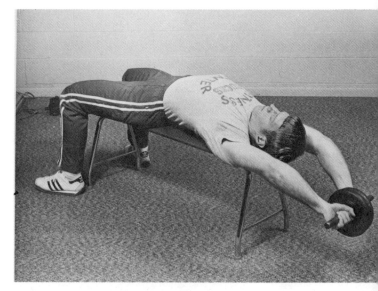

Figs. 35 and 36. the pull-over exercise is intended primarily to stretch and enlarge the rib cage rather than to build muscles.

especially, certain dumbbell exercises, or even push-ups. But to fully develop the chest, providing more room for the lungs to function, you need to expand the bony rib cage. This can be done with a simple exercise called the pull-over.

To do the pull-over, lie on the floor or on a bench, and hold a light weight (barbell handle, a pair of light dumbbells, or a dumbbell bar with a couple of small plates at the center) directly over your chest with your arms straight. Then lower the weight behind your head while inhaling high in your chest, holding your abdomen in. You should time the inhalation so your lungs are full just before the weight touches the floor (or reaches the full stretch permitted by your flexibility, if you are lying on a bench). You should feel your chest lift and stretch as your arms lower the light weight. Then bring the weight back up to the starting point, exhaling. Repeat 10 to 15 times.

Enough weight should be used in this exercise to provide a good stretch and give your muscles a little work so you don't get dizzy from hyperventilating (deep breathing without moving). The exercise also develops the chest muscles and the upper part of the latissimus muscles to some extent, but the idea is to stretch the rib cage, and no effort should be made to handle really heavy weights. You can get a good workout in the straight-arm pull-over with from 20 to 50 pounds. (If you're using dumbbells, the weight would range from a pair of 10-pounders to a pair of 25s.)

A bodybuilding exercise called the bent-arm pull-over is done similarly, but with arms bending freely and head hanging over the end of the bench. However, that is not within the scope of this book. The bent-arm pull-over is an advanced bodybuilding exercise for the chest and upper back muscles.

A tip for the beginning bodybuilder: If you want to enlarge your chest quickly, do a set of 10 to 15 deep-breathing, full-stretch, straight-arm pull-overs after each set of squats in your workout.

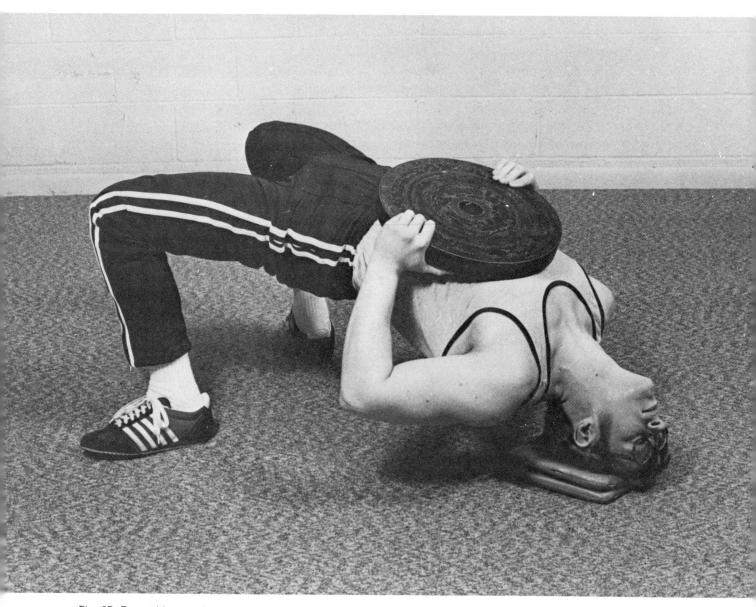

Fig. 37. Even without weights, the wrestler's bridge is a good way to strengthen neck muscles, but its effectiveness is increased by adding resistance as shown.

chapter 3
BASIC EXERCISES USING SPECIAL APPARATUS

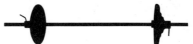

In addition to the basic barbell exercises already described, there are a number of other fundamental weight training exercises that call for additional pieces of apparatus. I will describe some of the more important ones briefly, especially some of the basic dumbbell exercises that you can do with no more equipment than one of the small barbell-dumbbell combination sets.

First, however, there is an exercise for your neck that requires only a folded towel or sweat shirt plus barbell plates of various weights. The exercise is the wrestler's bridge, so named because it is a defensive maneuver used by wrestlers and is also practiced extensively by wrestlers to condition their necks for the sport. Fold a towel or some other thick cloth several times to form a pad. (If you have access to a padded mat, additional padding probably won't be necessary.) Place the pad on the floor and lie on your back with your head at the near edge of the pad. Pull your feet up close to your buttocks, and arch your body up, digging your head into the pad by tensing your neck muscles. Arch all the way up so that you are supported by your feet and forehead. Return to the floor and repeat the bridging action eight to twelve times. When this feels easy, after a few workouts, hold a five- or ten-pound barbell plate on your chest and do eight to twelve bridges. The potential for neck strength is greater than you might imagine, but most people will not want to proceed beyond bridging with from 10 to 50 pounds of additional weight.

EXERCISES WITH DUMBBELLS

The press, rowing, curl, and pull-over exercises described earlier can be performed with dumbbells. In pressing and curling, especially, dumbbells are very effective because they force you to work equally hard with both arms. With a barbell, there is some tendency to do more of the work with your better-coordinated arm. You can't handle as much total weight with dumbbells as with a barbell, however, because they are somewhat harder to control. If you can press 100 pounds

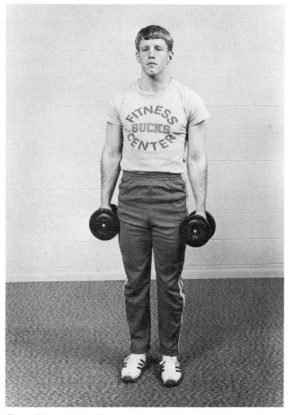 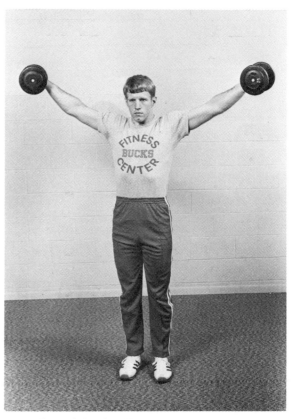

Figs. 38 and 39. The section of the deltoid muscles at the outer edges of the shoulders is strengthened by raising dumbbells directly to the sides. Note that the forward end of each weight is tilted down slightly at the height of the raise.

ten times on a barbell, for example, you may find it equally difficult to press a pair of 40- or 45-pound dumbbells the same number of repetitions.

The most important dumbbell exercises, because they can't be done satisfactorily except with dumbbells, are the various forms of raises to the sides. The lateral raise with dumbbells, which is unsurpassed for developing the outside part of the shoulder muscles (deltoids), is done as follows. Stand erect, feet a comfortable distance apart, and hold a pair of light dumbbells at your sides. Raise them simultaneously directly to the sides, keeping your knuckles up and level, to a point about even with your ears—somewhat higher than shoulder height. To keep your knuckles up and focus the work on the side part of the deltoids, make an effort to actually point the front ends of the dumbbells slight-

ly down at the highest part of the raise. Lower the weights smoothly under control, and do eight to twelve repetitions.

When doing lateral raises, you should keep your arms fairly straight, but it isn't necessary to keep your elbows forcibly locked. A slight unlocking of the elbows allows you to do the exercise more comfortably. This exercise should be done in three sets as you gain strength. Unloaded dumbbell handles are enough for most people to start with. If the handles alone feel ridiculously light, start with dumbbell handles loaded with 1¼- or 2½-pound plates. Strong men can do this exercise with 15-, 20-, 25-pound, or even heavier dumbbells, but most exercisers tend to loosen up a lot in the style of performance as the weights get much heavier than 25 pounds. I often wonder if it is the deltoid or the ego that is being developed as I see men

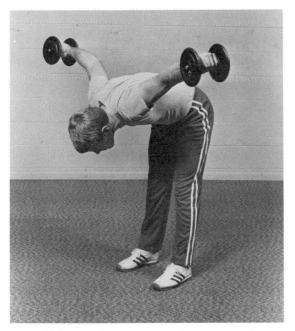

Fig. 40. To work the back section of the deltoid muscles directly, it is necessary to raise and lower the weights while leaning forward.

swinging 40- and 50-pounders up with arms bent almost to a right angle.

The lateral raise develops the sides of the shoulders, and all kinds of presses develop the fronts of the shoulders, but to develop the backs of the shoulders more than they are developed by such exercises as cleans and rowing, you have to perform the lateral raise while leaning forward to approximately a right angle so that the weights are raised up and back. Less weight may be used in this lateral raise than when doing the exercise standing. You may find it easier to hold good position if you place your head against an object to remind you to keep leaning at the same angle while you raise the dumbbells.

A variation of the lateral raise, done lying on a bench, is called flying because it is an inverted version of the motion made by a bird's wings. This is one of the best exercises for the pectoral muscles of the chest because it works them more directly and exclusively than the bench press does. To do this exercise, lie on your back (supine) on a bench and hold two dumbbells directly over your chest, arms slightly bent and knuckles out. Maintain the same arm bend throughout the exercise. Lower the dumbbells to the sides while inhaling. Then, while exhaling, bring the dumbbells back up in an arc until they meet over your chest at the starting position. This exercise, which should be done for eight to twelve repetitions, three sets, is for the chest, not the arms. If you keep your arms bent (to take strain off your elbows and shoul-

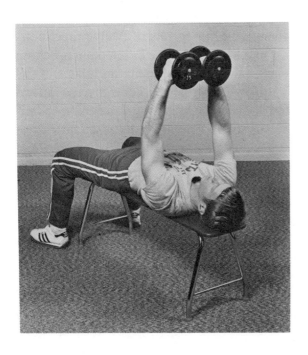

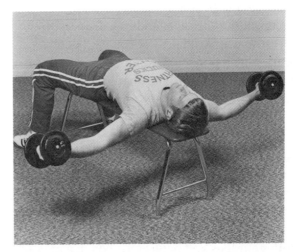

Figs. 41 and 42. The "flying" exercise is done with arms slightly bent to take strain off the elbows. This exercise focuses the work on the pectoral muscles of the chest.

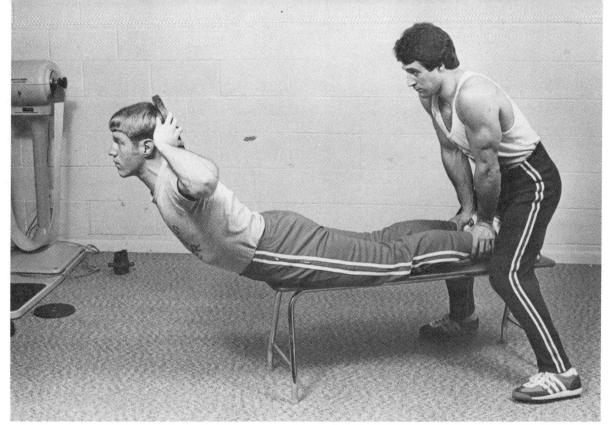

Fig. 43. Hyperextensions focus on the muscles of the lower back. The exercise is especially effective if a person holds a weight behind his head.

ders) but rigid, you can concentrate on raising the weights by contracting your chest muscles. Light weights, three to five pounds on each dumbbell, are enough to start with, but it is possible to work up to 25-, 30-, or 35-pound dumbbells or more. As with lateral rasies, some people lift heavy weights in this exercise, but the men tend to loosen up in the performance so that the exercise becomes a semi–bench press with dumbbells and strongly involves the arms and shoulders as well as the pectorals.

HYPEREXTENSION FOR THE LOWER BACK

Another important exercise that can be done with an ordinary bench and the help of a training partner, but is better done with special apparatus, is the back hyperextension. To do this exercise, lie face down (prone) with your legs and pelvis on a bench and your torso extending past the end of the bench. Your feet must be anchored firmly so you can raise and lower your torso in this posi-

tion, an exercise that is the best single way to focus on the muscles of the lower back (the lumbar area). You should do the exercise with your hands behind your head, arching upward as high as possible and then lowering your body so your forehead almost touches the floor. Perform eight to twelve repetitions. When two or three sets of twelve repetitions becomes easy, hold five or ten pounds behind your head and begin again at eight.

This exercise can be done more comfortably on special hyperextension benches available in gyms, but it is valuable no matter what kind of Rube Goldberg bench arrangement is used, providing the equipment is stable and safe. There would be a lot less lower back injury and discomfort if everyone would do hyperextensions and sit-ups two or three times a week, even without additional weight held behind their heads. One physical therapist found no lower back problems in people who could hyperextend with three times as much weight behind their heads as they could

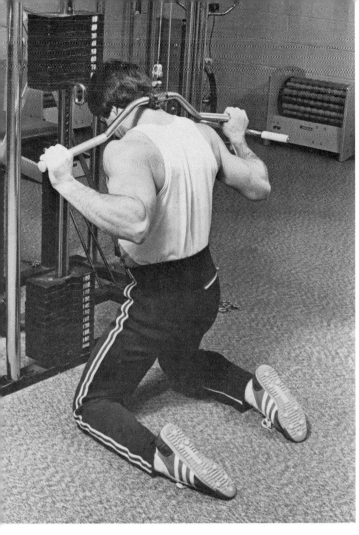

Fig. 44. The "lat machine" is one of the more useful items of accessory equipment for weight training. It permits the practice of chinning-type exercises with less than body weight and is especially effective for developing the latissimus dorsi muscles.

lift in sit-ups with knees bent. On the other hand, people who lacked this three-to-one strength ratio often had low back injuries. In other words, if you can sit up ten times with 10 pounds, you should be able to hyperextend ten times with 30 pounds. This ratio may be difficult to maintain as you develop abdominal strength, but some weight-lifting champions have done the hyperextension exercise with 200 pounds!

EXERCISE MACHINES WITH PULLEYS

Two types of exercise machines found in gyms are especially useful if you can gain access to them. One is the overhead pulley with a curved or bent handle, called a "lat machine." The name comes from the fact that pulling the handle down to your upper chest or to your shoulders at the back of your neck is a very good way to develop the latissimus muscles that give your back a V shape. Pulling a weight that limits you to ten repetitions for three sets, using a wide grip on the handle, is especially effective for widening your upper back. Chinning with a wide grip has the same effect but requires that you use your own weight, whereas on a "lat machine" you can begin with much less and work up gradually, using eight to twelve repetitions for three sets.

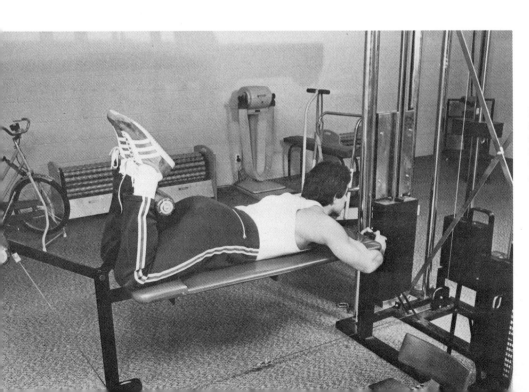

Fig. 45. Another useful accessory is the leg curl apparatus, which provides a means of directly exercising the hamstrings at the backs of the thighs.

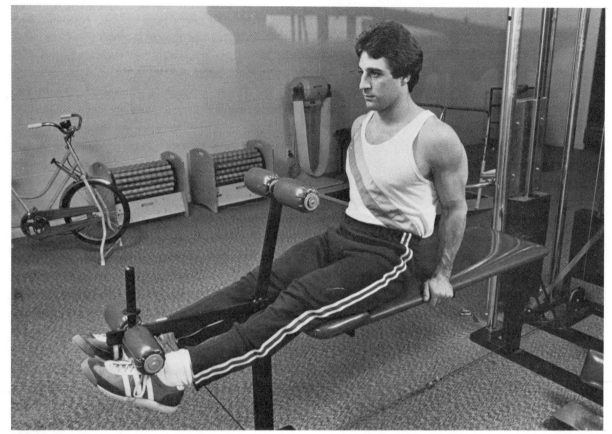

Fig. 46. Leg extensions, shown with a pulley apparatus, strengthen the quadriceps muscles and help stabilize the knees. This exercise is especially useful in rehabilitation, since there is little strain on the joint while the muscles are being worked.

Another machine that usually involves pulleys to a weight stack (with a pin to select the poundage) is one that works the muscles that bend and extend your legs. You develop the backs of the legs by lying prone on a bench, placing your heels against a padded resistance arm, and then flexing your legs to bring your heels as close as possible to your buttocks. This is a leg curl, and it develops the thigh biceps, or hamstrings. The same machine has another padded resistance arm that you use while lying supine or sitting. You place your insteps against it, then extend your legs to develop the muscles at the fronts of your thighs, the quadriceps. These exercises are valuable in stabilizing the knees to prevent injury or to rehabilitate them after injury. For both exercises, work progressively in three sets of eight to twelve repetitions.

THE INCLINE BENCH

A piece of equipment found in most well-equipped gyms is the incline bench, an exercise bench tilted at about 45 degrees or adjustable a few degrees on either side of 45. This type of bench is used for pressing with dumbbells and a barbell, for curls with dumbbells, and to maintain a firm position exercising face down (prone) in the lateral raise for the back part of the deltoids. Curling dumbbells on an incline bench isolates and stretches the biceps, but pressing on an incline is the primary use for the apparatus. The incline permits you to press straight up while working the front part of your deltoids and the upper part of your pectorals at about the angle a shot put or discus is delivered; so it is an especially useful piece of apparatus for weight men in track and field.

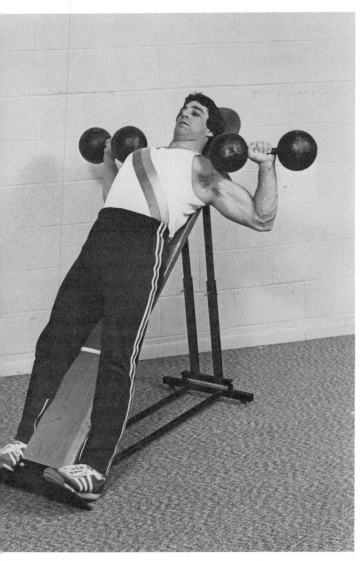 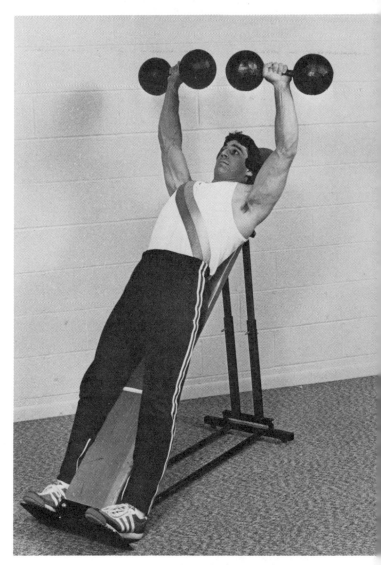

Figs. 47 and 48. Pressing on an incline, especially with dumbbells as shown, effectively strengthens the uppper chest, the front part of the deltoids, and the arms.

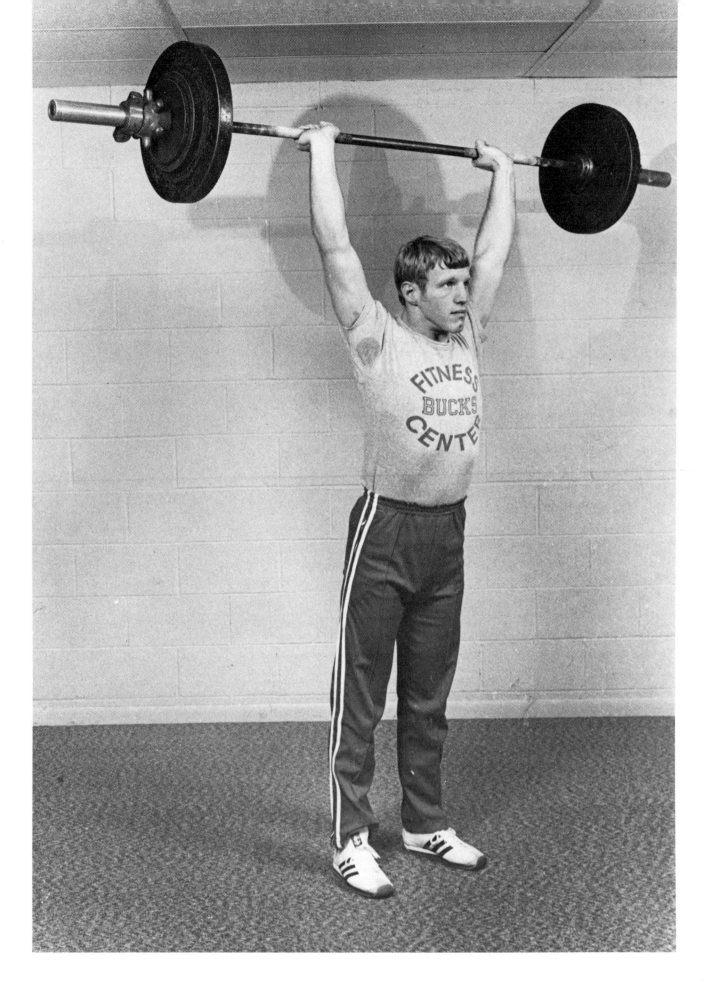

chapter 4
USING BASIC WEIGHT TRAINING

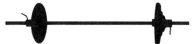

As I've been describing the strength-building exercises of basic weight training, I have covered a general, all-around approach (three sets of eight to twelve repetitions), an approach for building more strength and power (increasing weight with each set while decreasing repetitions), and a keep-fit approach (one to three sets of about ten repetitions with a moderate weight). I've also referred often to lifting done by champion athletes in sports other than weight lifting.

This section outlines some programs to show how the exercises can be organized into training routines. Percentages given refer to percent of best single effort. For example, if you can lift 100 pounds once in a clean, 65 percent would be 65 pounds, 85 percent would be 85 pounds, and so on. If you can lift 200 pounds, 65 percent would be 130 pounds, 85 percent would be 170 pounds.

GENERAL STRENGTH BUILDING AND CONDITIONING

Monday Wednesday Friday

Warm up with 20 to 50 sit-ups, two sets of five power cleans, and one set of eight overhead presses. The weights used for warm-up should be no more than 50 percent of the amount you can lift one time.

Power clean, 65 percent x 5, 75 percent x 3, 85 percent x 3, 90 percent x 2, and 95 percent to 102½ percent x single cleans.

Curl, three sets of 8-12.

Press, three sets of 8-12.

Squat, 50 percent x 10 and three sets of 8-12.

Pull-over x 10 after each set of squats.

Rise-on-toes, three sets of 10 to 20.

Rowing, three sets of 8-12.

Bench press, three sets of 8-12.

Tuesday Thursday

Jog 15 minutes, from one to two miles.

KEEP-FIT ROUTINE

In this routine, strength training is emphasized one week and jogging is emphasized
the next.

**Alternate Weeks, Monday Wednesday Friday
and Tuesday Thursday**

Sit-up x 20-50 repetitions.
Power clean 60 percent x 5, 75 percent x
5-10.
Curl, 60 percent x 10, 75 percent x 5-10.
Press, 60 percent x 10, 75 percent x 5-10.
Squat, 60 percent x 10, 75 percent x 10-15.
Pull-over x 10 after each set of squats.
Rowing, 60 percent x 10, 75 percent x 5-10.
Bench press, 60 percent x 10, 75 percent x
5-10.

**Alternate Weeks, Tuesday Thursday
and Monday Wednesday Friday**

Jog 10 to 20 minutes.

MUSCLE TONING FOR WOMEN

Three Days a Week

Sit-up x 10-20 repetitions.
Hyperextension x 10-15.
Squat x 10, two or three sets.
Pull-over x 10-15 after each set of squats.
Rise-on-toes x 10-20, two sets.
Sit-up x 10-20.
Curl x 10.
Bench press x 10.
Flying exercise x 10, one or two sets.

Three (Alternate) Days a Week

Walk briskly or ride bicycle 15 to 30 minutes
or alternately walk and jog 5 to 15 minutes.

Unless a woman is interested in competitive sports and actually needs a strength-train-
ing program, she need not use more than 15 to
50 pounds in the squat, rise-on-toes, curl, and
bench press exercises, and three to five pounds
on dumbbells for the flying exercise.

LIGHT PROGRAM FOR ATHLETES

This program is designed for athletes in sports
requiring minimal strength but great endurance, well-developed skills, or both.

Two or Three Days a Week

Sit-up x 20-50 repetitions.
Hyperextension x 10-20 (5 pounds behind
head).
Rowing x 8-12.
Squat x 8-12, two sets.
Bench press x 8-12, two sets.

Five or More Days a Week

Practice special conditioning or skills needed
for sport.

HEAVY PROGRAM FOR ATHLETES

This program is for athletes in sports where
strength and power are primary requisites.

Monday Wednesday Friday

Sit-up, x 20-50 repetitions.
Power clean, 65 percent x 5, 75 percent x 5,
80 percent x 3, 85 percent x 2, 90 percent x
1-3, occasionally continuing to 100 percent
or 102½ percent x 1.
Bench press, 60 percent x 8, 75 percent x 5,
80 percent x 5, 85 percent x 3, 90 percent x
1-3, occasionally continuing to 100 percent
or 102½ percent x 1.
Squat, 40 percent x 10, 65 percent x 5, 75
percent x 5, 85 percent x 3, 95 percent x 1-3,
occasionally continuing to 100 percent or
102½ percent x 1.
Pull-over x 10 after first and last sets of
squats.
Curl x 8-12 for 2-3 sets.
Lateral raise x 10 for 2-3 sets.
Rowing x 10+8+6 with increasing weights.
Press x 8+5+5+3+1 or 2 with increasing
weights.

Tuesday Thursday

For a track workout, jog an easy half mile, then walk the turns and run the straightaways at three-fourths speed or faster for a total of one-half to one mile of alternate walking and running. As the season approaches, football players should reduce the weight program to power clean, bench press, and squat, and reduce weights used to a maximum of 90 percent except when they feel unusually strong.

At the same time, increase running to meet coach's requirements (fast intervals for football efficiency; more or less distance running according to whether the coach stresses it). Wrestlers should also reduce the intensity of the strength training as they approach actual competition, except that they need much more running and should reduce the weights further, to 70-80 percent, as they increase their endurance work and practice on the mat.

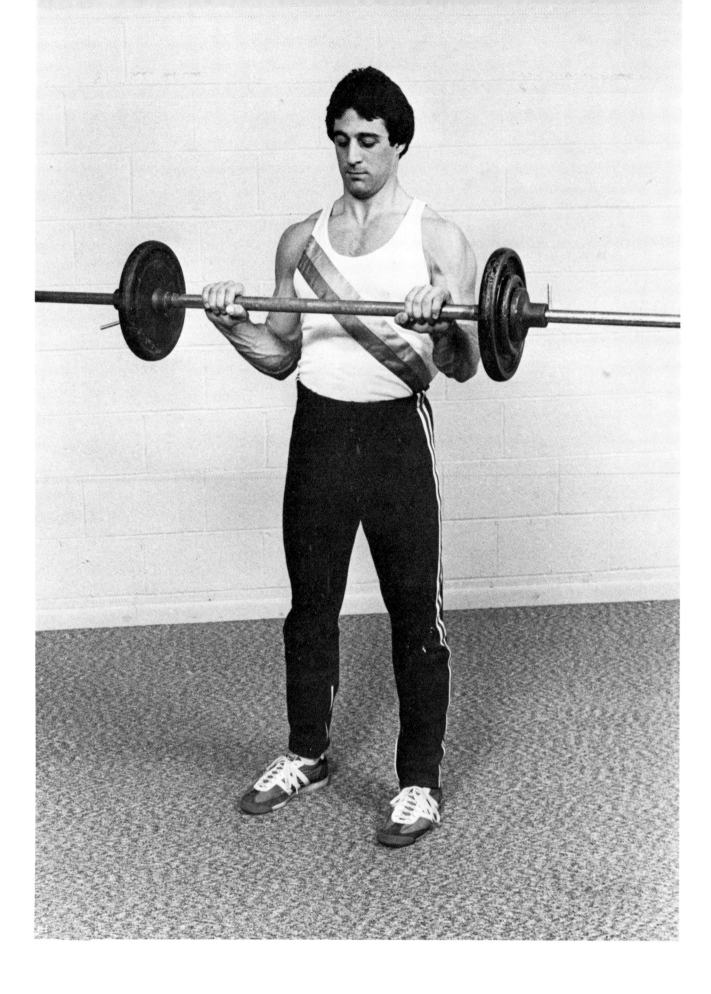

chapter 5
WEIGHT TRAINING FOR THE ATHLETE

One of the difficulties in attempting to prescribe training programs on the basis of the experience of outstanding athletes is that people with superior natural endowment tend to succeed regardless of what specific approach they use. The approaches I have settled on after many years of experience with strength training for athletes are based as much on the moderate (but highly satisfactory) success of relatively average people in sports as on the great success of the few unusually gifted people I have had the good fortune to work with. The programs I have outlined are not the only way to achieve good results. For one thing, I am concerned in this book only with broadly general approaches, not with special problems that may need somewhat different handling. But in general, a very basic approach to off-season strength training will work; I've seen it work with high school, college, and professional athletes. Clyde Emrich, a former 198-pound weight lifting champion who is strength coach for the Chicago Bears, uses essentially the same basic approach. Clyde can individualize the programs according to the players' needs, but he emphasizes power cleans, presses, and squats. The Bears' big starting linemen could power clean 300 pounds, and four of the strongest men on the team could bench press between 400 and 450 pounds. Emrich reported that Walter Payton, star running back, could easily power clean 240 pounds while weighing 205.

Weight training for athletic conditioning is often grossly overcomplicated. I have been guilty of this myself in the past, being influenced by the success of certain outstanding athletes who had their own favorite programs. After long experience with and observation of many fine athletes specializing in a variety of sports, however, I am convinced that specific details of different individuals' programs have little significance. Specific methods or specific types of equipment used to work muscles against resistance are much less important than the fact that the major muscle groups are exercised vigorously.

All athletes improve by adding strength,

and the extent to which their performance is helped by weight training depends upon (1) the need for strength and power in their sport and (2) the extent of the individual athlete's strength deficiency.

If a baseball player has adequate natural strength and is highly skilled, quick, and well coordinated, he has very little need for strength training. His sport does not call for great strength, but the advantage of strength can be seen in the success of strong players who are skilled and well coordinated and who can hit and throw the ball farther and faster than weaker players. Deficiency in strength is more apparent in sports that require more explosive power and sustained muscular efforts, especially football, wrestling, and the field events of track and field. Even in basketball, however, with its emphasis on skill, quickness, and endurance, added strength can provide a distinct advantage. Taller players, in particular, often need a strength program to provide the muscle required to move their large frames effectively. A basketball player needs power to jump well and to grab rebounds away from opposing players. The most effective way to add this strength is with a weight training program.

The weight training program of a basketball player can be much less intensive and time consuming than that of a football player, wrestler, or shot-putter, of course. But the practice of squats to near knee level and overhead presses is especially beneficial for increasing jumping power and rebounding effectiveness.

With regard to training athletes, one point worth emphasizing is this: Added strength improves the performance of a skilled athlete, but strength does not take the place of skill, especially in sports where skill is a prime requisite. And neither strength training (heavy resistance exercise) nor endurance training (running) can really make it *easy* for an athlete to perform at a high level in a specific sport. As long as the athlete is putting out a hundred percent, his efforts won't feel subjectively easy. If he is strong and fit, however, he will be more effective than he would be otherwise.

A major part of the conditioning for a sport is specific. What the strength and endurance training provide is the foundation to build on. The strong, enduring athlete can function at a higher level than one who relies on practicing the sport for his only exercise. Also, basic strength and endurance training minimize the risk of straining subpar muscles, including the heart. Furthermore, well-developed muscles help protect against impact injuries in contact sports.

Another important point: There are many instructors and equipment salesmen touting specific exercise systems and pieces of equipment as essential to athletic success. In view of this, it is well to remember that new methods and equipment have been coming on the scene for decades; while most have merit, none has proved to be indispensable. Almost all increase strength and thereby improve athletic performance. And most approaches and equipment are worth a try, though it is doubtful if any could possibly live up to advertising claims. The basic approaches and simple equipment described and pictured in this book have stood the test of time: they have been used successfully and effectively for the better part of a century. And they will provide anyone who is willing to work at them with all he or she needs in the way of strength training for athletic success and physical fitness.

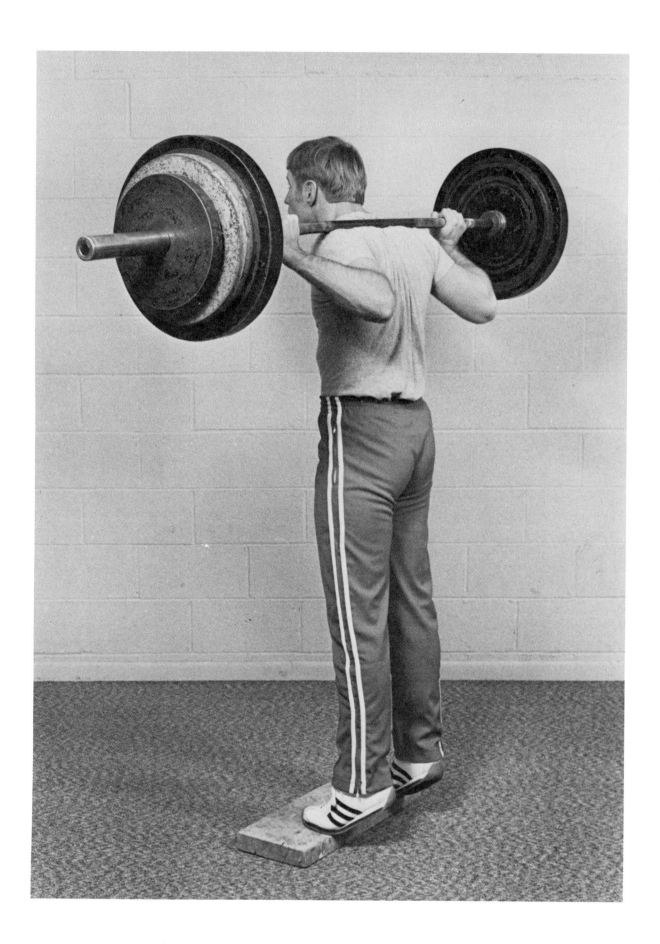

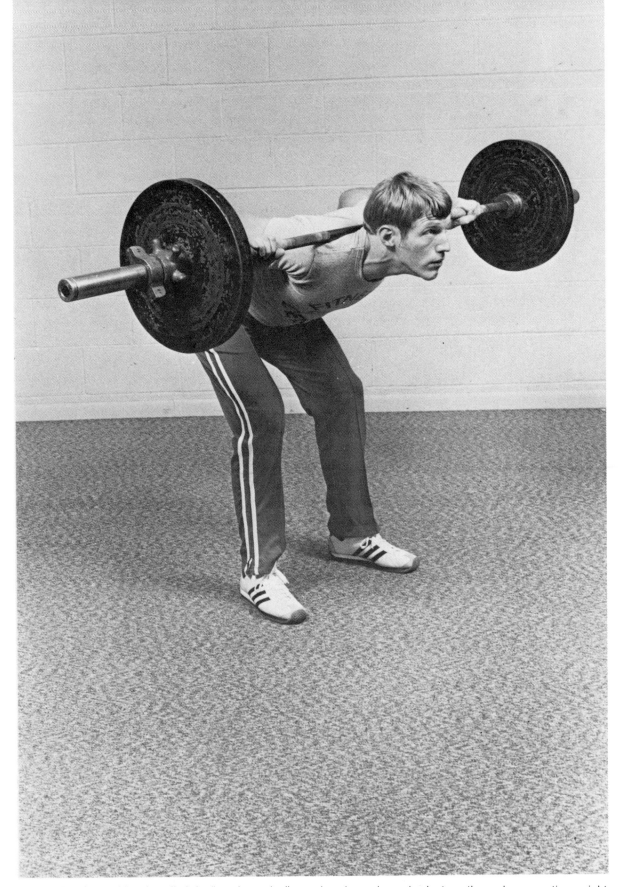

Fig. 49. The forward bend—called the "good morning" exercise—is used as a back strengthener by competing weight lifters. Note that the knees are slightly bent for this exercise.

chapter 6
WEIGHT LIFTING IN COMPETITION

There are actually two kinds of official international competition in which Olympic standard barbells are lifted. One is called Olympic lifting (and is part of the Olympic Games), and the other is called power lifting. The latter is something of a misnomer, because the two Olympic lifts—the snatch and the clean and jerk—are performed much more explosively—with power—than the ''power'' lifts. The latter come closer to being tests of unadulterated, grinding strength.

The power lifts consist of three of weight training's basic exercises, done with specific rules in single efforts to lift the greatest amount of weight possible. The lifts are the squat (with a requirement of bending the legs until the tops of the thighs are slightly below parallel, then rising); the supine press on bench (with a requirement of pausing briefly with the weight at the chest before pressing it); and the dead weight lift. Both strength and technique are important in becoming proficient at these lifts, and competition takes place in weight classes as Olympic lifting

does. For details about power lifting, read Terry Todd's book *Mastering Power Lifting,* published by Contemporary Books, Inc.

Olympic lifting began as a five-lift competition—two one-arm lifts plus the two-arm press, snatch, and clean and jerk. It later became a three-lift competition (the one-arm lifts were eliminated) and is now a two-lift competition. (The press was eliminated because its technique had become essentially the same as that of the jerk and it could not be officiated properly.)

Competition is divided into weight classes with the following limits, given in kilograms (kg) and pounds.

Kg	Pounds
52	114½
56	123½
60	132¼
67½	148¾
75	165¼
82½	181¾
90	198¼

100	220
110	242½
Over 110	Over 242½

Each lifter is permitted three attempts at each of the two lifts. He may select as much of an increase as he wants between the first and second attempts, providing he increases at least 10 pounds or 5 kilograms (11 pounds). He may also increase as much as he wants for his third attempt, providing he increases at least 5 pounds or 2½ kilograms (5½ pounds).

There are two exceptions to the increase requirements: (1) If the lifter fails, he may repeat the same weight (to a total of three attempts); (2) if he decides he wants to take only a 5-pound or 2½-kilo increase after a successful first attempt, he may do so except that he then forfeits his third attempt. A lifter may not drop back to take a lighter weight once the weight of the barbell has been increased.

The first of the two Olympic lifts is the snatch, in which the lifter is required to pull the weight from the floor all the way to straight arms overhead in a single unbroken motion. He must then stand erect with his arms and legs straight, feet on a line, and hold the weight under control, at which time the referee signals that he may lower it to the platform.

The second of the two lifts is the clean and jerk. In this lift, the athlete is required to pull the barbell from the floor to his chest in one motion (the clean) and then to shove it overhead in a second quick motion (the jerk). Again, he must hold the weight overhead under control with his arms and legs straight and feet on a line until the referee signals that he may lower it.

In lifting the weights, the athlete may use special techniques to lower himself under the barbell as he raises it. At one time, two techniques were used about equally for the snatch and the clean. Some lifters preferred the "split" technique and some preferred the "squat." With experience, and refinements of both techniques, it developed that the squat was the superior style, and today very few lifters employ the split except in the jerk, where the technique is appropriate and squatting would not be.

The official Olympic barbell is 2.2 meters (7 feet, 2½ inches) long overall and measures 1.31 meters (51½ inches) between the inside collars. This permits a wide hand spacing, which is especially necessary in the snatch. Taller lifters often use the widest possible grip. The barbell handle has a diameter of 28 millimeters ($1\frac{1}{10}$ inches), but the portions at the ends where the plates are slipped on are thicker, having revolving sleeves that turn easily and permit a smooth turnover at the end of the pull in the snatch or clean. The largest plates, weighing 25 kilograms (55 pounds), 45 pounds, or 20 kilograms (44 pounds), are 45 centimeters in diameter, which is 17½ inches. It isn't possible to duplicate the dimensions exactly with an exercise set, but you can practice Olympic lifts on a 6-foot exercise bar by placing the collars 48 inches apart and using 50-pound plates.

There are three aspects to learning the two Olympic lifts: (1) developing pulling and pushing power, (2) mastering the form, and (3) putting the form and power together.

THE WARM-UP

Before beginning a training session of Olympic lifting, it is important to warm up carefully. This will help you function more efficiently and, even more important, will help prevent injury. In actual competition, you will be required to wear a neat T-shirt and trunks or an official lifting suit, like those worn by lifters in contests pictured in this book. But in training, you should wear a sweat suit or warm-up suit of some type. You may wear the warm-up suit over your lifting costume when you are not actually on the platform for an official lift.

Begin your warm-up by loosening up with some easy bending and stretching, leaning

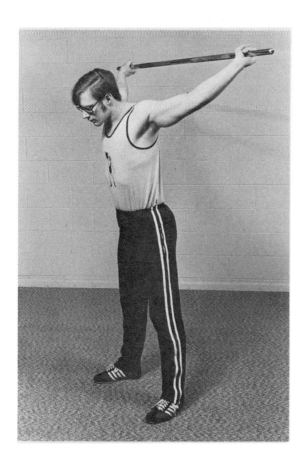

Figs. 50 and 51. Stretching exercises for the shoulders and legs are important in warming up, to minimize the danger of "pulls" and strains.

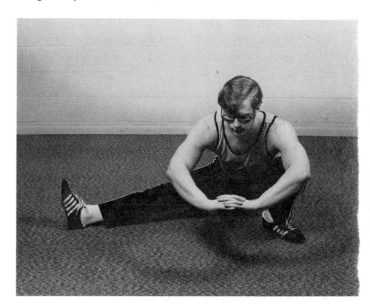

from side to side, rotating your upper body from the hips and waist, and bending to reach the floor with knees slightly bent. Then take an unloaded bar or a very light weight (an unloaded Olympic bar weighing 44 or 45 pounds is plenty) and press it overhead a few times, first from the chest and then alternately from the chest and from low at the back of the neck. Next place the bar across your shoulders and, with knees slightly bent, bend forward from the hips a few times, stretching your hips and back. Then squat a few times with normal foot spacing, with feet close together, and with feet wide apart. For additional back strengthening, as well as a warm-up stretch, you can add weight and (carefully) perform the forward bending exercise three sets of five repetitions. This is called the good morning exercise because it is like a bow. Strong lifters handle body weight and more—but proceed with caution to avoid back strain.

To stretch your shoulders, hold the bar overhead with hands wide apart—as wide as you would hold them for the snatch lift. Lean forward slightly, and rotate the bar back from your shoulders several times. Give your legs some additional stretching by squatting, thrusting one leg out to the side, and shifting from leg to leg in a one-legged squat position without rising.

The sit-up and hyperextension exercises described in the section on basic weight training are good ones to include in a warm-up, though weight lifters should strive to handle progressively heavier weights in the hyperextension. Ten to 20 pounds is plenty to use for fitness, but champion lifters practice hyperextensions with 100 pounds and more. (Incidentally, when you warm up for a contest, it isn't necessary to do any sit-ups or hyperextensions.)

After warming up, proceed to the lifts or exercises planned for the day. Begin your heavy exercises by doing one light set or by doing the lift with light weights at less than full speed and then at full speed. For example, if you plan to do squats with weights ranging from 200 to 400 pounds, you should take a warm-up set of five to ten repetitions with a much lighter weight, ordinarily 132 or 135 pounds (which is the weight of an Olympic barbell with two 20-kilogram or 45-pound plates). If you plan to do squat snatches with weights of 200 to 250 pounds, you should go through the motions with an unloaded bar and with 135 pounds before moving up to the sixty percent and heavier weights.

Most young lifters are impatient with warming up and with practicing form with very light poundages, but this is exactly the way David Rigert, the 198-pound world champion, began his workouts. Rigert went through the motions with 45, 65, and 95 pounds, then worked in the 115, 135, and 200 range before moving on carefully to training poundages of 300-plus in the snatch and 400 plus in the clean and jerk.

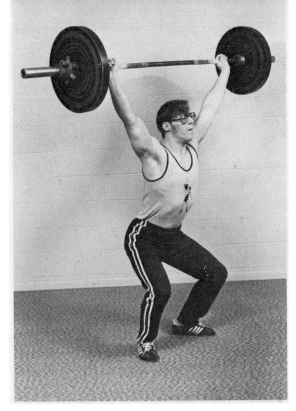

Fig. 52. This is the height of the pull for the power snatch. The exercise is done like the power clean, shown earlier, but with a wider grip and an all-the-way-up pull. The knees are bent as shown to catch the weight overhead.

TRAINING FOR THE SNATCH

For Olympic lifting in the squat style, you need shoes with built-up heels. Shoes made specifically for weight lifting are advertised for mail-order sale in the leading magazines covering the sport, such as *Strength & Health* and *Iron Man*. But you can begin to practice Olympic lifting wearing athletic shoes or even work shoes with the heels built up by a shoe repairman. The height of the heel may not exceed four centimeters, which is 1⅝ inches; be sure to observe this limit.

To learn the squat snatch position, take an unloaded barbell handle or a broomstick, hold it overhead with a relatively wide hand spacing (taller men should put their hands about four feet apart), and practice sinking into the squat position while holding the bar overhead. This will require more or less shoulder flexibility, depending upon how erect you can "sit" in the deep squat position. All lifters need to get the bar back and

their head forward, and they must hold their body in an erect, back-flat position. If you allow your back to round, your arms will unlock and the weight will come down.

In addition to learning the deep squat position with the bar overhead, you should be training on flip snatches, or power snatches. These are done like the power clean, described earlier in the section on basic exercise, except that you use less weight and pull the barbell all the way to arms' length overhead.

Do the power snatch like this. Get set close to the barbell, feet approximately hip-width apart and toes projecting past the bar. Crouch and take an overhand grip, as in the clean, but with a hand spacing that would be wide enough for you to assume the deep squat position with the barbell overhead. Keep your hips lower than your shoulders and your back arched in or flat, not rounded. Let your arms hang loosely straight and lift by extending your legs and back, keeping the weight close to your knees and thighs. As the bar reaches the point in front of your thighs from which you can pull best, pull hard with your arms, continuing to extend your legs and back, thrusting your hips forward as the barbell passes your chest and face. At this point, bring your elbows under the barbell and ram your arms to full lock overhead. There should be enough impetus from the pull that there is no perceptible pause and push to straighten your arms. In competition, you may not turn your wrists over until the bar has passed the top of your head, so it is advisable to pull the bar at least this high in performing power snatches, in order to learn a proper high pull. In essence, you pull the weight all the way from the floor to arms' length overhead.

As you bring your arms under the weight in the power snatch, you should also be dipping at the knees (possibly jumping your feet slightly sideways at the end of the pull) and bringing your body down and forward to fix the weight at straight arms with your head slightly forward.

The Squat-Style Snatch

The pull for the squat-style snatch is the same, except that with weights too heavy to pull all the way up, you lower your body to a squat position under the barbell while straightening your arms overhead. This action requires lots of practice with an unloaded bar and with light weights. You must learn to pull the weight approximately chest high and then, as you rise on your toes to get the ultimate leg impetus into the lift, you jump your feet to the position you have found is most comfortable for you in the deep squat. As you jump, you pull yourself down under the weight, not turning your wrists over until the bar has passed your head. Thrust your head forward as you quickly lock your arms with the weight overhead.

Balance is critical as you catch the weight overhead in the squat position, because the weight tends to push you deeper into the squat, and you must control the barbell and rise immediately. You cannot allow the weight to be too far front, so you must jump under it—but not too far or it will crash behind you. Only practice can give you the proper feel for this position and teach you to find it in the split second you have before the barbell starts down.

To learn the lift, practice power snatches, practice the form with an empty bar and then with increasingly heavy weights, and practice full squats with the weight held overhead as well as with the barbell across your shoulders. You may need training partners to help you get the weight into position for squats with the barbell overhead. Once you can lift more weight in the squat style than you can power snatch, it is no longer necessary to work on squats with the weight overhead. Front squats and regular squats will provide all the extra leg work you need.

As you get the feel of the lift (which may take weeks, incidentally, so don't be discouraged if you make progress only slowly), you can begin to think about some of the finer points. You can never completely master them by training alone, or with other inexperienced lifters, or by reading books and articles. You will have to find experienced lifters to train with you and—if you're lucky—a good coach. But you can teach yourself to pull close and accelerate the weight upward from thigh level.

The pulling style has evolved more and more into a two-stage effort in which there is minimal acceleration from the floor to thigh level and then an explosive second pull from the thighs upward. After thoroughly mastering the second pull acceleration, you can begin to speed up the first pull, being careful not to deviate from correct position or lose power in the follow-through of the second pull. A common mistake of beginners is to

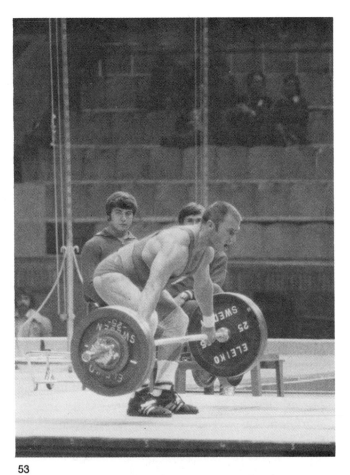

53

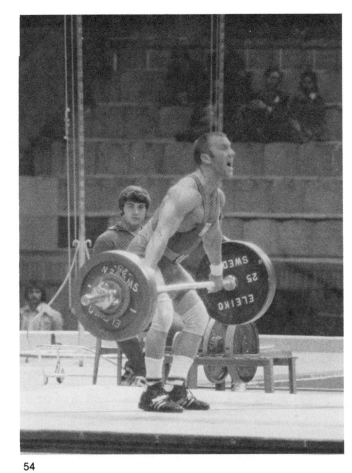

54

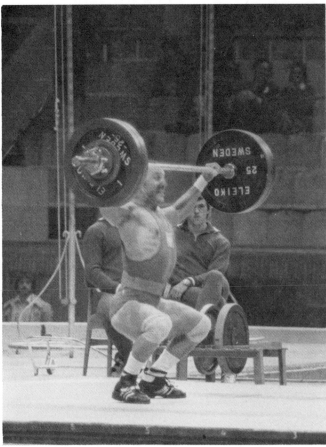

55

56

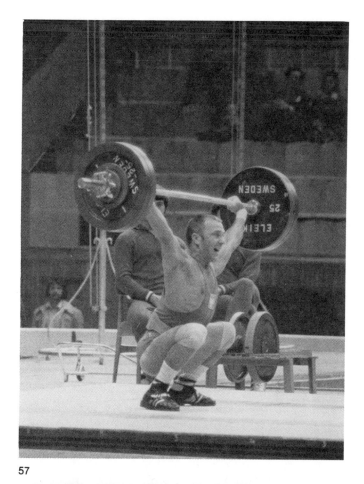

57

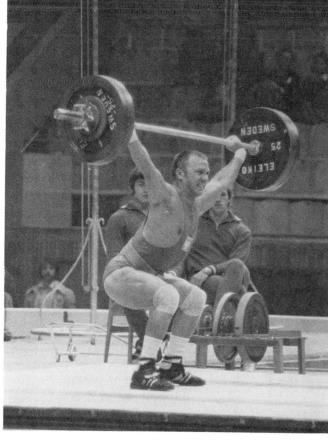

58

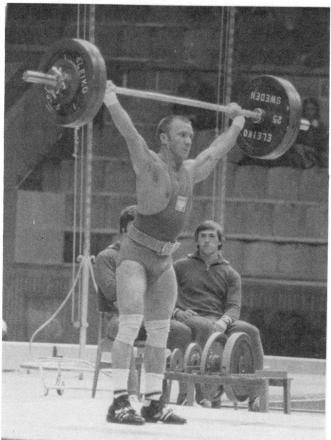

Figs. 53–59. This series shows Zbigniew Kaczmarek, one of the world's best 148-pound lifters, snatching 303 pounds—more than twice his own weight. Note that he lifts exactly as this book describes the pull. Hips are lower than shoulders and back is flat at the start. An explosive acceleration leads to full leg and back extension at the height of the pull. Then, in the fourth photo, he jumps under the barbell, pulling himself down to catch it at straight arms, and rises immediately to hold the weight under control and await the referee's signal to lower it.

pull hard from the floor and then fail to follow through with acceleration from thigh level.

Many lifters employ a pronounced "double dip" action very quickly when pulling in the snatch and clean, rebending their knees slightly as the barbell reaches the bottom of their thighs, to get a strong leg drive into the top part of the pull.

In teaching yourself to keep the bent-knee position and get the bar close to your thighs, you should remember that a clearly evident stopping of the barbell at the thighs can result in disqualification. It is most unfortunate that there are technicalities in officiating that are not interpreted uniformly by officials. As I mentioned earlier, you should thoroughly familiarize yourself with the official rules. You should also attend weight-lifting contests to see how the lifts are actually performed and what the judges will and will not pass.

For preliminary training on the snatch, you can break up your workout as follows. First practice power snatches, all-the-way-up pulls. Begin with a light weight—at most, about 50 percent of what you can power snatch once—and do five repetitions. Then add weight in ten- and five-pound increases until you can only do two repetitions or a single lift. For example, do 50 percent x 5, 60 percent x 3, 70 percent x 3, 75 percent x 3, 80 percent x 2 or two singles, 85 percent x 1 or 2, and 90 percent x 1. About once every week or two, work up to a limit and try to establish a new percentage basis for the series.

While training on the pulling exercises, and when lifting heavy weights in the snatch and clean, you may find that you can hold the barbell handle better if you employ a hook grip. This simply means that you wrap your forefingers or first two fingers around your thumbs as you grip the bar. Hooking definitely helps secure your grip for the pull, but some lifters take their thumbs out of the hook after cleaning a weight and before jerking it. Some go so far as to place their thumbs behind the bar, with their fingers, before jerking the weight overhead.

After completing a series of power snatches, practice the squat snatch form—pulling the bar up and dropping into the deep squat position—with no disks on the bar. Then, as you become comfortable with the deep squat position, begin to work up to about the same poundages you can pull up in the power snatch. When you become comfortable with such weights, you should be ready to work up to considerably more—an increase of about 10 to 20 percent. For example, if you can power snatch 100 pounds, your squat snatch limit might be 120. Or, if you can power snatch 180 pounds, good form should enable you to squat snatch 200 to 220 pounds.

Once you have mastered the squat form so well that your best squat snatch is distinctly superior to your best power snatch, you can work up on the squat-style lifts with a percentage system. First warm up carefully by going through the motions with an unloaded bar and some very light weights. (World superheavy champ Alexeyev would warm up with the bar, then with 65, 95, and 115 pounds before proceeding to heavier weights when he could snatch more than 400 pounds.) Then power snatch 50 percent of your best squat snatch once and squat snatch it two or three times. Proceed to 60 percent for three squat snatches, either touching the barbell lightly to the floor or pulling the repetitions from thigh level (called pulling from the hang). Move on to 70 percent for three repetitions, 75 percent for two or three, 80 percent for one or two, and 85 percent to 90 percent for three to five single lifts. Once a week, or every other week, try to increase your single lift personal record by 5 or 10 pounds. Then readjust all the weights for your training lifts, based on percentages of the new personal best.

A third aspect of training for the snatch is to work for additional strength and power.

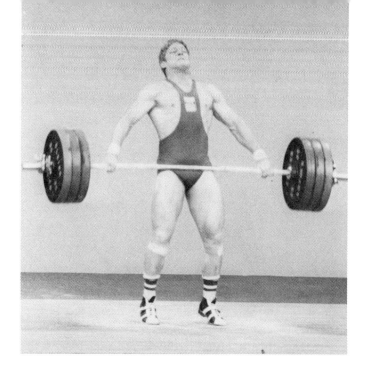

Figs. 60–62. This sequence shows Lee James, silver medalist at 198 pounds in the 1976 Olympic Games, snatching 363 pounds. Note that after he finishes his leg drive and rises on his toes with the full extension, he jumps his feet slightly sideways to a position that is comfortable and strong for him to catch the weight overhead in the squat from which he rises to hold the weight and receive credit for the lift. Compare these pictures with the side view of Kaczmarek doing the same lift.

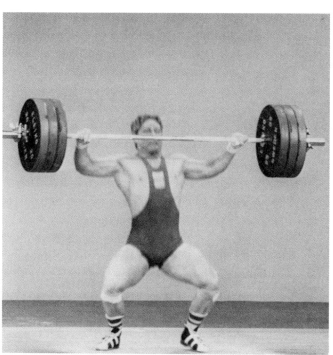

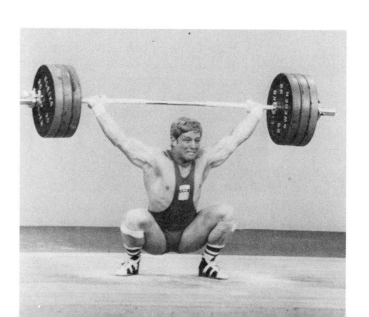

After completing power snatches and squat snatches, load the barbell to approximately what you lifted in your best single effort in the squat snatch. Then perform high pulls with the same wide grip that you use for snatching. The pull should be done exactly as if you were actually going to snatch the weight, except that you pull the bar up to touch your chest and then lower it either to the floor, to just below your knees, or to your lower thighs for three to five repetitions. In this exercise, you should make no effort to drop under the weight; instead, concentrate on pulling high, only leaning forward slightly at the height of the pull to touch the bar to your chest. You should soon be able to high pull from 10 percent to 20 percent more than you can lift in the squat snatch, doing three to five repetitions with each weight. Work up to as much weight as you can pull to the bottom of the chest muscles; this should be considerably more than you can snatch and about as much as you can power clean.

After completing the pulls, stand erect, hold the barbell so it hangs across your thighs, and shrug your shoulders several times, attempting to touch your shoulders to your ears. Do three sets of five to eight repetitions of this exercise, called the shrug.

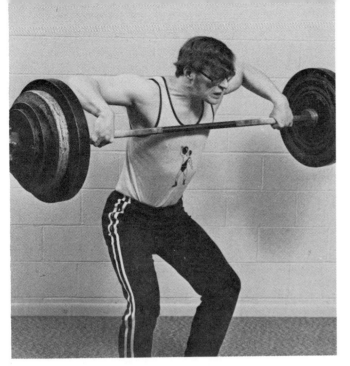

Fig. 63. Pulling power is developed by hauling heavy weights chest high, as shown. The pull is started exactly as if the weight were going to be lifted overhead, but the barbell is pulled only to the point shown.

The Split-Style Snatch

It is easier to pick up rudimentary form in the split-style snatch than in the squat, though ultimately you should be able to lift more in the squat. The split-style is like the squat except that at the height of the pull, as you rise on your toes in making the final effort, you thrust one leg forward and the other back, each foot moving about the same distance. A right-handed person usually thrusts the right leg back. Cock the forward leg as you pull yourself under the weight, so that you land with your front leg in a flexed position and your rear leg extended back almost straight, just slightly bent. The front foot should land flat, with the knee at about a right angle and slightly forward of the ankle. The rear foot strikes the floor in an on-toes position. Once under the weight, whip your hands over and ram your arms to full lock smoothly, with no obvious press-out, rocking deeper on the front leg in a one-legged squat position. As soon as your arms are straight, rise by straightening both legs, and then step forward to bring your feet on a line, holding the weight overhead

under control. You must not allow the knee of your rear leg to touch the floor, because this is cause for disqualification.

THE CLEAN AND JERK

Most of the training for the clean and jerk is divided to focus on the pull and push portions separately. But occasionally it is necessary to try the complete lift to determine how much you can do and to accustom yourself to the recovery and second effort that is required for the jerk after having completed a difficult clean.

Practice for the clean is much like that for the snatch. First do power cleans, then practice the full squat clean, and finally do clean-grip high pulls and squats with the weight held at the chest in the clean position and (using heavier weights) with the weight on your shoulders.

The power clean is done as described in the basic exercise section. In training for competitive lifting, however, you should emphasize the fine points of the pull more than when doing the lift strictly as an exercise. Focus on a smoothly controlled lift from the floor to thigh level and then on getting the bar close to your thighs and accelerating more pronouncedly from your thighs to your chest. Try to hold a bent-knee position through the first part of the lift or to rebend your knees quickly without stopping the upward progress of the barbell as you get into the second pull acceleration. The best way to learn this is by deliberately moving slowly during the initial lift to thigh height, then concentrating on explosive acceleration all the way from the thighs to the chest. Once you have mastered the follow-through of the second pull, you can begin to accelerate sooner, from the floor, as long as you do not yank at the resting barbell. You must move the weight off the floor with the big muscles of your legs and back, then try to accelerate. If you try to accelerate too much in the early part of the pull, you will be unable to follow through properly. It often seems as though a hard yank from the

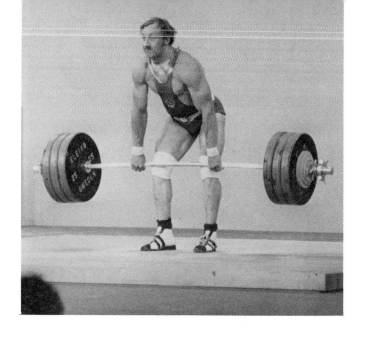
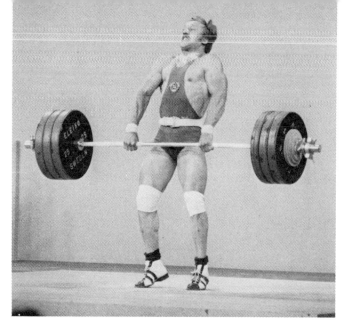
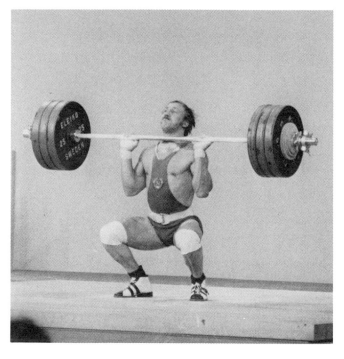
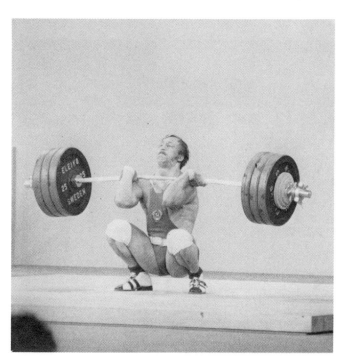
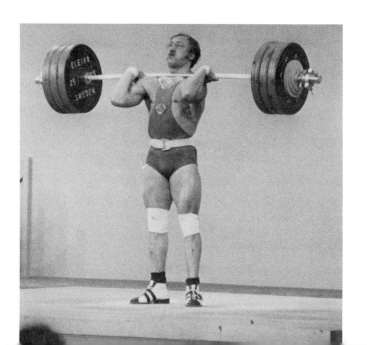
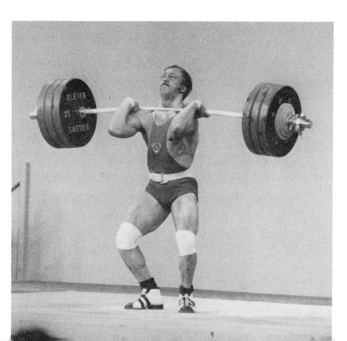

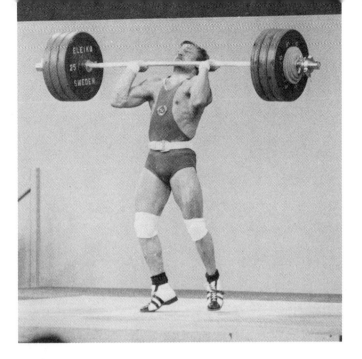

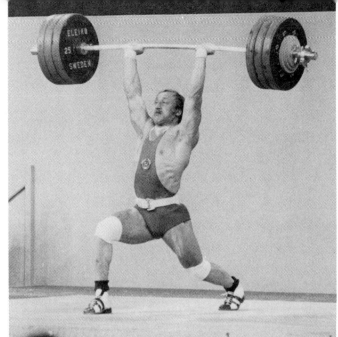

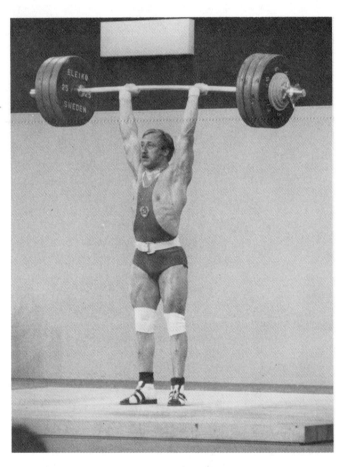

Figs. 64-72. This sequence shows Valeri Shary, world 181-pound champion, cleaning and jerking 424 pounds. The first photo shows him just getting into his pull, the second one nearly full extension. In the third picture he is jumping under the weight, just about to recieve the barbell on his chest; in the fourth the mass of iron forces him to rock bottom in the squat. He rises immediately and gets set for the jerk, dips at the knees and drives the weight straight up, again getting good extension from his legs before jumping into a fore-and-aft split to get under the barbell. The final photo shows him holding the weight under control, awaiting the referee's signal to lower it. Note Shary's unusual technique of switching from a hook grip to place his thumbs behind the bar as the weight turns over and is about to strike his chest. This is not recommended for anyone with less than superhuman coordination.

floor will provide enough impetus for the weight to "coast" to your chest. In fact, you can do this with lighter weights, but doing so will only teach you a bad habit that will cause you to fail with heavier weights.

For doing repetitions, lower the weight to the tops of your thighs, still standing erect and with your arms hanging straight. Then lower the weight farther by bending your knees and leaning forward from the hips, keeping your back arched in. Try pulling the weight back up from high on your thighs, from half-way down the thighs, and from just above your knees. Experiment until you find the point from which you can pull most strongly. This is the point at which you should try to accelerate and "explode" into the second pull when you are lifting a weight from the floor in a snatch or clean.

When practicing the power clean to train for lifting, begin with about 50 percent of what you can power clean once and do five repetitions. Then add weight in 10- and 5-pound increases until you can only do one or two. For example, do 50 percent x 5, 60 percent x 3, 70 percent x 3, 75 percent x 3, 80 percent x 2 or 3, 85 percent x 1 or 2, and 90 percent x 1 or 2. Once every week or two, work up to your limit to try to establish a new percentage basis for the series.

The Squat-Style Clean

As in training for the snatch, practice form for the squat-style clean with an unloaded bar and light weights. The pull for the squat clean is the same as that for the power clean, except that you do not pull the barbell as high. The pictures showing the squat clean (Figs. 73–79) show that world class lifters pull the bar only a bit higher than their waists. Then they jump down under the weight, continuing to pull as they jump. This continuing pull has the effect of pulling them down into the squat position.

Briefly, then, in the squat clean you pull the barbell approximately waist high and jump under it, turning your hands over and thrusting your elbows forward and upward to fix the weight across your upper chest and shoulders. Keep your elbows high, because it is against the rules to allow your elbows or arms to contact your legs in the clean. (It could also be painful to allow your elbows to strike your knees as the barbell pushes down against your hands and wrists.)

Catch the weight at your chest before reaching the deepest squat position. Then control the weight, keeping an erect position,

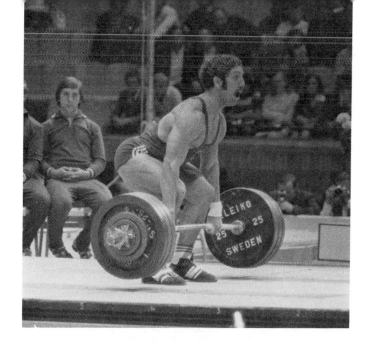

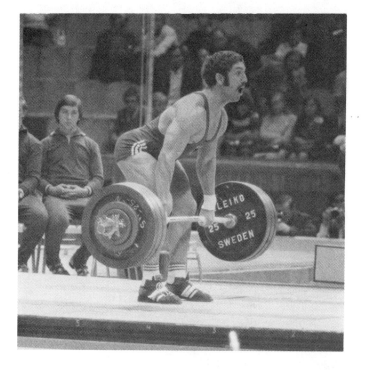

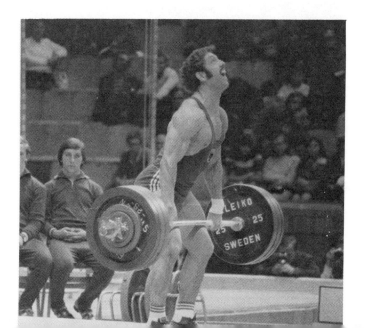

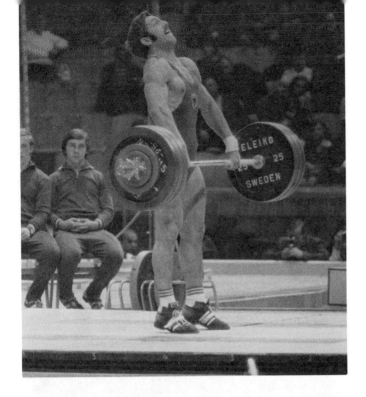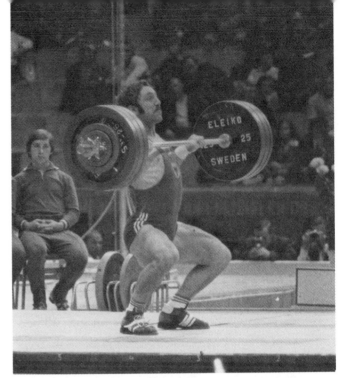

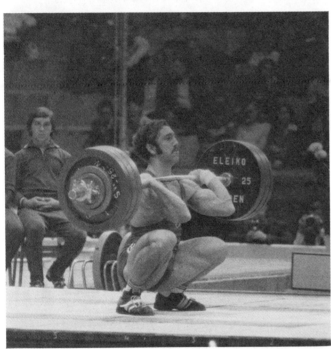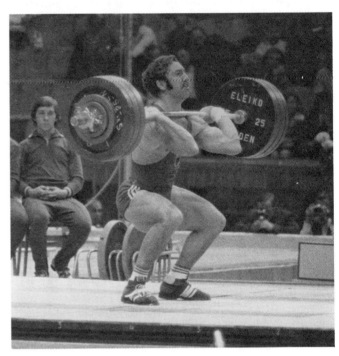

Figs. 73–79. Rolf Milser, one of the world's best 181-pound lifters, is shown cleaning 441 pounds. His position is exemplary as he keeps his hips low, back flat, and knees bent until he explodes into the height of the pull with full extension. Then he jumps under the weight, pulling himself down to catch it on his chest and control the barbell in a deep squat, keeping his elbows forward and high above his knees. As soon as he hits bottom, he starts up, still holding his back straight and his elbows high.

as it forces you into the lowest squat position. It is important to drive up out of that deep squat immediately, taking advantage of the full stretch of the muscles and rebounding quickly, or the weight will either defeat your effort to rise or make it so difficult that you will have no strength left to complete the jerk. Keep your elbows high as you rise from the squat, keep your back arched—not rounded, and ease your hips forward as you push up out of the deep squat position.

In competition, you would gather your resources to jerk the weight overhead after rising from the squat clean, but in training, you lower the weight to your thighs or below your knees for additional repetitions. Work patiently with light weights to master the squat clean form, and then build up gradually until you can squat clean more than you can power clean. The deep squat clean takes a lot of energy, so with heavier weights you will want to do fewer repetitions than for the squat snatch or the power-style lifts. Begin with 50 percent of your best clean and do three. Then do 60 percent x 3, 70 percent x 2, 75 percent x 1 or 2, 80 percent x 1 or 2, and 85 percent to 90 percent x 3-5 singles.

As in training for the snatch, you should also practice pulling weights high from the floor, using poundages you cannot actually clean. Start with about what you can lift in your best clean, and, using the same handspacing as for the clean, pull the weight as high as possible for three repetitions. Try to touch your chest with the bar. Add 20 pounds and do three more pulls. Add another 10 or 20 pounds and do two or three more. Keep adding poundage until you can no longer pull the weight above belt level.

After completing the pulls, practice shrugs —three sets of five to eight repetitions. Stand erect with arms straight as you grasp the weight. Shrugs strengthen the trapezius muscles running between your neck and your shoulders. These muscles add great impetus to your pull in the snatch and clean.

The Split-Style Clean

Cleaning with a split involves the same pull as for the squat except that you drop under the weight with the same leg action as described for the split snatch. Pull the weight as high as possible, as with a power clean, and then jump one foot forward and the other back. Land with the front foot flat and the front leg cocked at approximately a right angle. The back foot lands on the toes, and the rear leg is almost straight. It is important

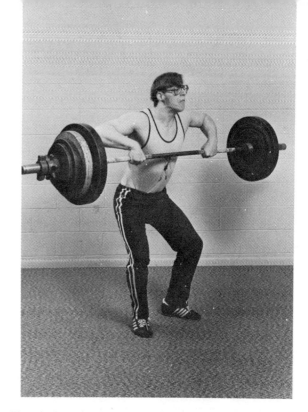

Fig. 80. Chest-high pulls, using the same grip as for the clean, are an excellent way to build strength and power.

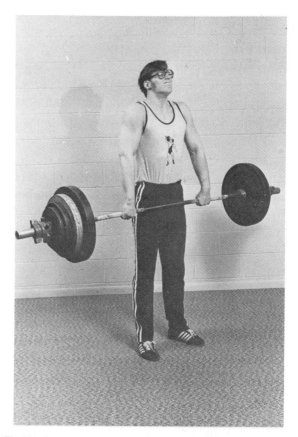

Fig. 81. Shrugs, in which a lifter attempts to touch his shoulders to his ears, should be done with the clean grip, as shown, and also with the wide grip used for the snatch.

to keep your front leg cocked so that your foot stays behind your knee; otherwise, you could not reach the low position you need with heavier weights. With the knee forward, you can sink lower and catch weights that are not pulled quite high enough. (But do not let your rear knee touch the floor.) In rising from the deep split, push up and back with the front leg before stepping up with the rear leg to get set for the jerk.

Jerking the Weight Overhead

The overhead portion of the clean and jerk calls for explosive power and total body and limb strength. After cleaning the barbell to your chest, hold it firmly across your collarbones and the front of your shoulders, keeping your elbows forward so the bar cannot slip down on your chest as you start the jerk. Get set with your feet on a line, a comfortable distance apart—about hip width. Then apply force with your legs, quickly bending and straightening your knees with an explosive but relatively shallow dip to drive the barbell straight up, holding your head back so the bar can pass. Follow through with a thrust from your arms, and jump off the floor at the end of the leg drive, sending one leg forward and the other back. During the jump, push yourself down under the weight as you push the barbell up. Land with the forward leg cocked at nearly a right angle, the rear leg almost straight, and the rear foot on its toes. Most right-handed people thrust the right leg back.

A description of the jerk with a splitting action may seem complicated, but look at the pictures; it's a relatively simple technique. If you develop good form in the jerk, you will only have to thrust the barbell upward to approximately the height of your head.

You need strength from the soles of your feet to the tips of your fingers to hold the weight overhead in the split position and then recover by straightening both legs partially and then stepping forward with the rear leg to bring your feet on a line. You must hold the weight overhead under control, with your feet on a line, to gain the official's approval before setting it down. As you lower the barbell to your chest, cushion the shock by resisting with your arms and bending your knees.

A few words about setting the weights down. The rules require that the barbell be lowered, not dropped, and at one time a lifter would be disqualified for allowing the weight to crash to the platform. Today, "lowering" seems to mean that the lifter must keep his hands on the barbell as he lets it drop, rather than merely walk away and let it fall where it may. The difference is insignificant, since the weights crash to the platform anyway. A training session of world class Olympic lifters makes a boiler factory sound like a quiet rest home by comparison, for every weight from 45 to 450 pounds is casually dropped from overhead or from chest height to bounce once or twice before coming to rest. These pampered champions must save their strength for lifting the weights and do not deign to waste energy lowering them.

A beginner training at home can't be dropping weights, however, and most clubs frown on your breaking up expensive lumber and bending Olympic bars that cost more than $100. So if you find yourself getting to the point where you can win a national championship and become an international contender, you may want to find a club where no one objects to having weights dropped with only token "control."

Training for the jerk involves building power by doing presses (some bench pressing, but mostly overhead presses), power jerks (or jerk-presses), and about three sets of five quick little quarter squats with the barbell held at your chest. The quarter squats should be done with about 10 to 20 percent more than you can jerk. The weight should feel heavy, but not so heavy that you can't bend and straighten your legs quickly, with a bouncy motion. And, of course, training includes work on form and technique.

Pressing to build power for the jerk should

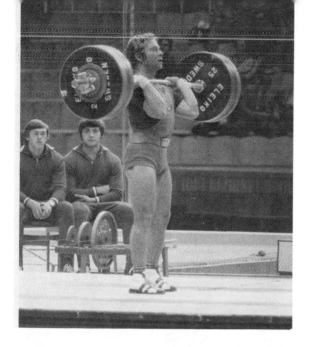
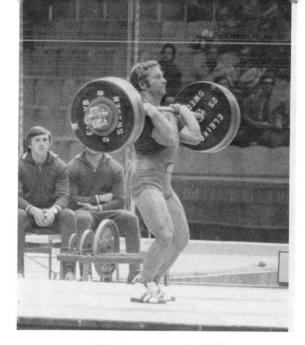
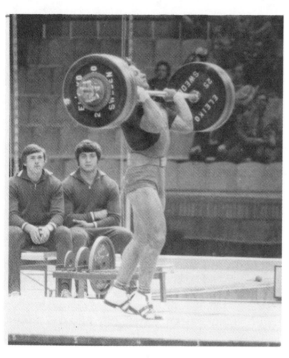
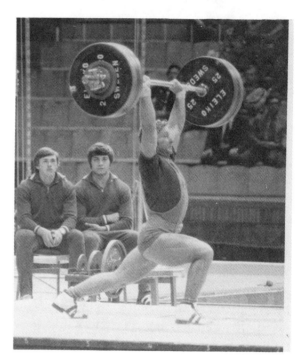
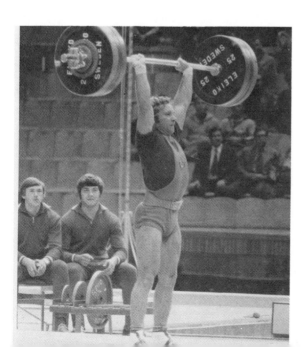

Figs. 82–86. Piotr Korol, a leading international 148-pound lifter, is shown jerking 391 pounds. After squat cleaning the barbell, he dips to drive the weight straight up. After fully extending his legs, he thrusts his right leg forward and his left leg back, landing in the split position as he rams his arms to full lock. You can see, from the head of the spectator in the background, that the barbell is not lifted quite as high as Korol's head for him to be able to get under it. In the final picture Korol holds the barbell under control until the referee signals that he may lower it.

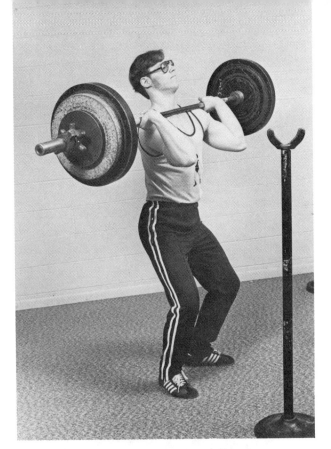

Fig. 87. This photo shows how far to bend the knees when driving the barbell upward in the jerk press, or power jerk. To gain added power, dip this low in quick, bouncy partial squats with heavier weights held at the chest.

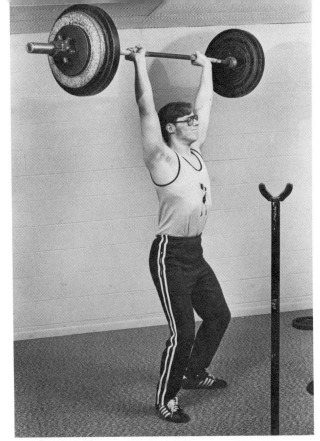

Fig. 88. A knee bend is used, as shown, to catch the weight overhead in the power jerk. The legs are bent once and fully extended to "kick" the weight upward, then bent again to fix the barbell overhead before finally straightening.

be done with few repetitions (5-3-3-2-2-1) and increasing weights. With a weight that you can only press once, do one or two additional overhead lifts by "kicking"—quickly bending and straightening your knees—to get the barbell moving. As you work up to still heavier weights, you will need to employ a second knee bend, about a one-quarter dip, to get under the weight as it goes up. You may also find yourself jumping your feet sideways a bit as you dip under the weight, as in the power clean.

It is important to learn the coordinated leg and arm drive of the jerk-press because it is the essence of the lift. It teaches you to drive the weight overhead, and after you have developed the power to jerk-press (or power jerk) 20 to 50 pounds more than you can press, you should be able to handle an additional 20 to 50 pounds by splitting. So continue to work for additional weight in the

power jerk, doing sets of two repetitions until you can complete only one.

Then drop back to a weight you can press easily, perhaps 50 to 60 percent of your best power jerk, and practice the split jerk technique, again working up in ten- and five-pound increases until you reach a weight that is fairly difficult to lift, about 80 to 90 percent of the amount you could lift with an all-out effort. Decrease the repetitions as you add weight: 3-3-2-2-1. Repeat three to five single jerks with the final weight.

For these training lifts, take the weight from squat racks at shoulder height, rather than cleaning each one, and replace the barbell on the stands after completing the jerks. If you are going to do a large series of lifts, your training will be much more efficient if you separate the cleans and the jerks. About once every two weeks, however, you should take a workout in which you warm up carefully and perform a series of snatches with increasing weights to a limit lift, followed by a similar series of cleans and jerks. This will help you determine how much weight you should be lifting in training and will also give you the feel of how you must perform the lifts in competition.

In training on the lifts, you should be aware of the reasons for disqualification, so as not to learn any bad habits. Lifts may be turned down by the officials (a chief referee in front of the lifting platform and two judges, one on either side) for the following reasons:

1. A perceptible break in the pull of either the snatch or the clean. For example, a person may fail to smoothly lift the barbell all the way up in one motion in the snatch, but instead use a pull-and-push motion. Or, during a clean, a person may touch the bar to the body at some point below the upper chest and then bring it to the upper chest with another effort. In either lift, stopping the barbell at the thighs and then starting it again is prohibited; this is called lifting from the hang.

2. Touching any part of the body except the feet to the platform. Such a violation is most likely to be a knee touch in the split-style snatch, clean, or jerk, but the buttocks may touch the floor in the squat style of lifting if the lifter is exceptionally flexible.

3. Starting a lift and then setting the weight down, providing the barbell is pulled as high as the knees.

4. A noticeably uneven straightening of the arms in either the snatch or jerk, or an incomplete straightening of the arms. Also, a lifter will be disqualified if he straightens his arms, then bends and restraightens them as he is bringing the barbell under control.

5. In the clean, touching the knees or thighs with the elbows or upper arms while in the squat position.

6. In either the clean or the snatch, touching the barbell to the thighs with a visible stop (in essence, cleaning or snatching from the hang). This does not mean that the bar may not touch the thighs, but merely that it may not perceptibly stop there. However, using grease or oil on the thighs to facilitate continuing movement is prohibited.

7. After a person cleans the barbell, he is allowed only one attempt to jerk it. Any apparent effort—such as a quick bending of the knees—counts as an attempt.

8. In both lifts, the weight must be held under control until the referee signals it may be lowered, and then it must be lowered and not dropped. Release of the bar with one or both hands before the barbell reaches the platform is considered "dropping" the weight.

9. While lifting, the lifter must stay within the ample limits of the platform, which is four meters square (more than twelve feet on each side). If he steps off the platform while attempting to lift the barbell, he will be disqualified.

For a detailed description of the weight-lifting rules, send $3.00 for an official handbook on weight lifting to the Amateur Athletic Union of the United States, 3400 West 86th Street, Indianapolis, IN 46268.

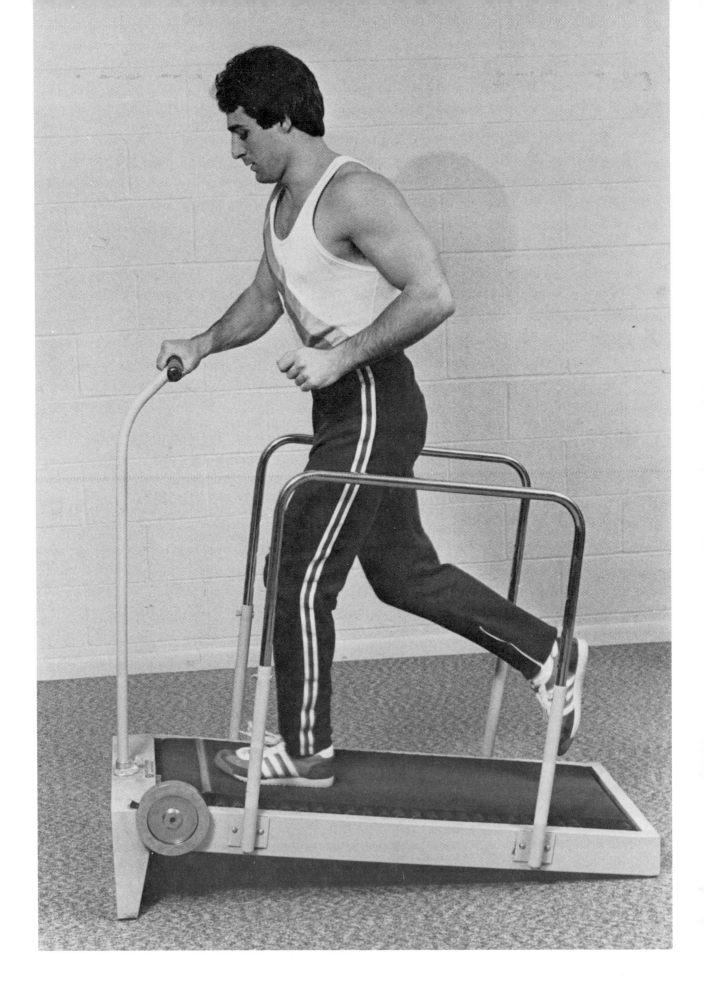

chapter 7
PLANNING A TRAINING PROGRAM

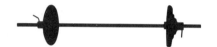

We have covered a basic approach to training on the Olympic lifts individually, but it is also important to plan workouts that integrate these individual parts into an overall program. If you tried to do, in one workout, all the training that I've described for the snatch, clean, and jerk—including the assistance exercises, you would soon become exhausted, or at least stale and overtrained. The workouts must be broken up into manageable work loads, and the total amount of work must be cycled so your body can recuperate and move on to greater heights.

For example, you might establish a three-day-a-week approach as follows (this program is scheduled Monday, Wednesday, and Friday; but you could train Monday, Wednesday, and Saturday; or Tuesday, Thursday, and Saturday):

Monday

Warm-up
   Power snatch, 5-3-3-3-2-1
   Squat snatch, 3-3-3-2-1-1-1-1

High pull, snatch grip, 3-5, 3-5, 3-5
Shrug, snatch grip, 5-5-5
Press, 5-3-3-2-2-1
Squat, weight overhead (until you can squat snatch more than you can power snatch), 5-5-5
Regular squat, 8-5-5-3-3-1

Wednesday

Warm-up
   Power clean, 5-3-3-3-2-2-1
   Squat clean, 3-2-2-2-1-1-1-1
   High pull, clean grip, 3-3-3-3
   Shrug, clean grip, 5-5-5
   Front squat, 8-5-3-2-1
   Bench press (for arm and shoulder strength, to help hold heavy weights at straight arms), 5-5-3-3-2-2-1

Friday

Warm-up
   Power clean, 5-3-3-2-1-1
   Press, 5-3-3-2-2-1

Power jerk, 2-2-2-1-1
Jerk (with split), 3-3-2-2-1-1
Quarter squat, weight at chest, 5-5-5
Regular squat, 10-8-6-4-2

A beginner, learning to do the lifts and simultaneously building strength, may follow the above program with the percentages given in the section describing the exercises and lifts. After two or three months, however, it will become necessary to arrange your workouts in cycles. It is necessary to plan cycles from workout to workout, from week to week, and from one part of the year to another. It is especially important to plan a training cycle in relation to a target date when you plan to enter a meet. Just before that date, you need several days of relatively easy training. It is absolutely foolhardy to do any lifting at all for two days before a meet. It is almost as bad to take a heavy or even a moderately heavy workout three days before a meet. In the last workout before competition, you should not handle more than 60 to 70 percent of the weights you plan to attempt in the meet; you should only reinforce positive neuromuscular patterns by performing successful lifts with weights you can handle easily. The last time you should handle even 90 percent of the weights you hope for in the contest is a full week earlier.

One of the first times a cycled approach was published in easy-to-understand form— in terms of percentages of best previous lifts —was in an article that John Terpak wrote for *Strength & Health* in the early 1950s, describing an approach he had used in coaching a Mexican national team. Terpak was one of the world's best middleweight (165-pound) lifters and a perennial U.S. champion during the 1930s and 1940s. He also was a superb split-style technician and analyst whose ability as a coach for competitive lifters was second to none. Since Terpak described a progressive percentage system some twenty-five years ago, such cyclic approaches have been refined so much that world-class lifters plan a full year's training to culminate with a top performance at a world or Olympic championship.

THE TRAINING CYCLE

A number of aspects of training must be considered in planning cycles. One is the total amount of work performed: the amount of weight lifted in every practice lift and assistance exercise multiplied by the number of times the lift or exercise is repeated. Another is the intensity of training. Sometimes you may not include a lot of assistance exercises in a workout, but instead practice lifting with heavy weights exactly as you would warm up and lift in a contest. The total amount of work may be less than in an all-around build-up workout, but the intensity of effort is so great that the session is highly fatiguing anyway. It is important not to push yourself too hard in both total work and intensity at the same time; if you do, it will be difficult for your body to recover, and you may find yourself going stale, unable to lift as much as in previous workouts.

During the buildup phase of training, strive to add a repetition, an exercise variation for a specific weak point, a set, or a few more pounds to a lift or an exercise. If one aspect of your training seems to stagnate, try to improve in another. Analyze your weaknesses, and concentrate on assistance exercises that help overcome them. If your second pull is not progressing, do more power cleans and high pulls from the thighs. Or set the barbell on blocks or boxes to force yourself to pull in your problem area. If the first part of your pull seems weak, do pulls with weights that you can lift only from the floor to belt level. If your recovery from the squat clean is weak, push yourself to handle heavier weights in front squats, holding the barbell at your chest. For the most up-to-date training approaches for special problems, you must associate with other good lifters and compare notes, and read articles on training approaches and special techniques in publications like *Strength & Health* and *Iron Man*. There you will find analytical articles by experienced coaches, men like Carl Miller and former world champion Tommy Kono.

As you reach the height of the buildup phase in your training, emphasize intensity: strive for heavier poundages in both training lifts and selected assistance exercises. Also, begin to reduce the total amount of work. For example, if you have been doing both shrugs and pulls on snatch and clean days, eliminate snatch pulls and clean-grip shrugs. Eliminate the bench press and, later, cut back on overhead presses. But continue to try for heavier weights or an extra repetition in practicing the snatch, clean, and jerk.

During the two weeks before a contest, reduce assistance exercises to an absolute minimum, test yourself on the lifts, and concentrate on technique. Allow your muscles and nervous system to recuperate so that you will be eager to try your limit in competition. Such tapering off before a meet is absolutely necessary if you hope to do your best in the contest. There is always the temptation to try yourself out repeatedly so as to reassure yourself that you can really hoist the weights that you plan to lift in competition. But don't do it! The usual result of such folly is that your best lifts are done in the training room. Too frequent limit efforts can leave you mentally and physically tired, too drained to perform well despite the stimulus of competition.

The following workout schedules show how a four-month training program might be planned to cycle through a buildup phase the first three months and then week-by-week training the month of the contest. A beginner planning to enter a novice meet in his district could use this type of approach, and it is also suitable for a more experienced lifter getting ready for a series of contests. For a series, the sequences for the final month or two weeks could be repeated, depending on the scheduling of the contests.

The workouts are based on the same three-day-a-week training approach outlined for learning weight lifting. This is certainly not the only way a program can be arranged, but it is workable for a lifter with no special problems. More advanced lifters develop such great strength and recuperative power that they frequently train four or five days a week, especially during the buildup phase.

HOW MUCH SHOULD YOU LIFT?

I have frequently alluded to lifts of 400 and 500 pounds by champions, but you are probably wondering how much you should be able to lift in order to consider entering competition. Early in your training, you should set a goal of being able to power clean your own weight plus 10 or 20 pounds. When you can do that, you will be strong enough to snatch almost as much in the squat style, with good technique, and to clean and jerk 20 to 50 pounds more, using the squat-style clean. At this point, if you are interested in becoming a competitive lifter, you should join the AAU and enter one or more novice meets. You won't disgrace yourself in such meets if you can snatch a barbell weighing 10 or 20 pounds less than your weight and clean and jerk 10 to 30 pounds more than your weight. If you're lucky, you might even win a trophy. Only by entering competition, and by observing more advanced lifters in action, can you really understand what it's all about.

Competition should stimulate you. It will give you "butterflies" in your stomach and other manifestations of nervousness, but it also provides additional stimulation, and you may find that you can outdo yourself under pressure. In early meets, try your previous personal bests on second attempts. You may find you can exceed them by 5 or 10 pounds on your third tries. Or, if nervousness causes you to miss on the second attempt, you can take the same weight again for your third try. When you can snatch 20 to 50 pounds more

	FIRST MONTH	SECOND MONTH	THIRD MONTH
	Monday	*Monday*	*Monday*
	Power snatch, 80–100%	Power snatch, 70–80%	Power snatch, 70%
	Squat snatch, 70–80%	Squat snatch, 80–95%	Squat snatch, 80–100%
	High pull, snatch grip, 100%	Shrug, snatch grip, 100%	Shrug, snatch grip, 100%
	Shrug, snatch grip, 100%	Press, 80–100%	Press, 80–90%
	Press, 80–100%		
	Squat, 70–80%	Squat, 70–80%	Squat, 70–80%
	Wednesday	*Wednesday*	*Wednesday*
	Power clean, 80–100%	Power clean, 70–80%	Power clean, 70%
	Squat clean, 70–80%	Squat clean, 80–95%	Press, 80–100%
	High pull, clean grip, 100%	High pull, clean grip, 100%	Squat clean, 80–100%
	Shrug, clean grip, 100%	Front squat, 80–100%	High pull, clean grip, 100%
	Front squat, 80–100%		Front squat, 80–100%
	Bench press, 80–100%		
	Friday	*Friday*	*Friday*
	Power clean, 70%	Power clean, 70%	Power clean, 70%
	Press, 70–80%	Press, 80–100%	Squat clean, 80–100%
	Power jerk, 80–100%	Power jerk, 70–80%	Clean and jerk, 80–100%
	Jerk, 70–80%	Jerk, 80–100%	Jerk, 70–90%
	Quarter squat, weight at chest, 100%	Squat, 80–90%	Squat, 80–100%
	Squat, 80–100%		

FOURTH MONTH

First Week	*Second Week*	*Third Week*	*Fourth Week*
Monday	*Monday*	*Monday*	*Monday*
Power snatch, 70%	Power snatch, 70%	Power snatch, 80%	Power snatch, 70%
Squat snatch, 80%	Squat snatch, 90%	Squat snatch, 90%	Squat snatch, 75%
Shrug, snatch grip, 90%	Squat clean, 90%	Shrug, snatch grip, 90%	Power clean, 70%
Press, 80%	Front squat, 90%	Press, 90%	Squat clean, 75%
Squat, 80%		Squat, 90%	Jerk, 75%
Wednesday	*Wednesday*	*Wednesday*	*Wednesday*
Power clean, 70%	Power clean, 70%	Power clean, 80%	Power snatch, 70%
Squat clean, 80%	Power jerk, 90%	Squat clean, 90%	Squat snatch, 70%
High pull, clean grip, 90%	Jerk, 90%	High pull, clean grip, 90%	Power clean, 70%
Front squat, 80%	Squat, 90%	Front squat, 90%	Clean, 70%
			Jerk, 70%
Friday	*Friday*	*Friday*	*Saturday*
Power clean, 70%	Power snatch, 70%	Power clean, 80%	Contest, 100% plus
Press, 80%	Snatch, 100%	Press, 90%	
Power jerk, 70%	Clean and Jerk, 100%	Power jerk, 90%	
Jerk, 80%		Jerk, 90%	
Squat, 80%		Squat, 90%	

than you weigh and clean and jerk 50 to 100 pounds more, you should surely have been able to win a novice meet and place or win in more advanced competition.

As examples of lifts that were good enough to place in novice meets, consider the following. At a novice meet in California, the 123-pound class winner snatched 137½ pounds and cleaned and jerked 192½. A beginner who cannot approach these lifts may be discouraged from entering, but he should not be; the third-place trophy in that class was won with lifts of 77 for the snatch and 110 for the clean and jerk. In the same meet, the 165-pound class was won with 154 for the snatch and 214½ for the clean and jerk. The 220-pound class was won with a 165-pound snatch and a 209-pound clean and jerk. In a major open novice meet on the East Coast, the 114-pound class winner lifted 55 in the snatch and 85 in the clean and jerk. (Women often place in these smaller weight classes, usually because there are no men, or only young boys, entered.) The 123-pound class was won with a 115-pound snatch and a 170-pound clean and jerk. A very good novice won the 132-pound class with 185 for the snatch and 235 for the clean and jerk, outscoring the 148-pound winner who lifted 180 and 220. The 198- and 242-pound winners had identical winning lifts of 220 and 280, but the third-place winner at 242 scored 175 and 205.

There are also contests with age limits. The national 148-pound title for sixteen and seventeen year olds has been won with 209 in the snatch and 264 in the clean and jerk. A national 165-pound title for ages eighteen and nineteen was won with 220 and 286. In a central states teenage meet, the 148-pound class was won with 185 and 235—excellent lifting—but second place went to more average lifts of 100 and 155. The 165-pound champion scored 160 in the snatch and 205 in the clean and jerk, better than the heavyweight (242), who lifted 135 and 190.

In major contests, too, there are often wide discrepancies between what it takes to win and to place. Sam Walker won the superheavyweight class (over 242) in a Dallas championship with the excellent lifts of 300 for the snatch and 400 for the clean and jerk. Walker was not only a superheavyweight but also a super all-around athlete who was the first schoolboy to put the 12-pound shot past seventy feet, later an international-caliber competitor with the 16-pound shot, and one of America's best lifters in the heavier classes. So it is not surprising that no one in Dallas could beat Walker. The second-place trophy was won with a 210-pound snatch and a 265-pound clean and jerk, however; so it is evident that the presence of an outstanding individual champion should not in itself deter other lifters from entering a contest. In that same Dallas meet, the 165-pound class winner scored a very good 235-295, but second place went to a 140-pound snatch and a 190-pound clean and jerk.

At one open meet in western Pennsylvania, the 242-pound class was won with a snatch of 185 and a clean and jerk of 200. On the other hand, at an open meet in eastern Pennsylvania, Bruce Klemens (who took the fine pictures of lifting sequences in this book) made very good lifts of 285 for the snatch and 365 for the clean and jerk, but placed only third in the 242-pound class against very tough competition.

These random examples of the lifts made to win and place in various classes at meets in different parts of the country are not given to compare the quality of lifting, but to show that there is a wide range in what it takes to win and place from one meet to another. And they are given to encourage the lifter who may think he is unworthy because he can't snatch a barbell equal to body weight, or perhaps even make a clean and jerk of more than body weight. If you pick your competition realistically, a body-weight clean and jerk is not a bad lift.

At the highest level of competition, however, it's another story. To compete successfully at the national level, and to hope to make an international team, you need to be able to snatch about 75 to 125 pounds more than body weight and to clean and jerk approximately 175 to 225 pounds more than you weigh. If you hope to place among the top three in a world or Olympic 114- or 123-pound championship, you must lift about 110 to 120 pounds more than body weight in the snatch and 175 to 200 over your weight in the clean and jerk. To place high in the larger classes, except the superheavyweight (unlimited) class, you must snatch about 135 to 185 pounds more than your weight and clean and jerk 200 to 280 more than you weigh. The superheavyweights, who generally weigh about 300 to 350, snatch 50 to 120 pounds more than they weigh (380 to 420 pounds) and lift 150 to 200 pounds over their body weight in the clean and jerk (490 to 550 pounds). Super athletes like Valeri Shary

(181 pounds) and David Rigert (198 pounds) have lifted 175 to nearly 200 pounds over their body weight in the snatch, and 260 to 285 over body weight in the clean and jerk. Clearly, a snatch of body weight plus 200 and a clean and jerk of body weight plus 300 are possible.

The following table shows a classification system used to rank weight lifters. From the table, you can see that a middleweight (165-pound) lifter could gain a Class IV rating by snatching 25 pounds less than he weighed, 140, and cleaning and jerking 15 pounds more than body weight, 180, for a 320-pound total. A heavier man, at 242, would need proportionately less for Class IV: a 170-pound snatch and a 220-pound clean and jerk would total 390. If you can make any combination of lifts adding up to a Class IV rating, consider entering novice competition. You need to score Class I or Master to compete successfully at the national level, and world class lifters all rank as Elite.

Olympic Lifting Qualification Standards
(total on two lifts)

Rating	114	123	132	148	165	181	198	242	Unlimited
Class IV	245	260	275	295	320	335	350	390	405
Class III	285	305	320	345	370	395	410	455	470
Class II	350	370	385	410	450	480	500	550	570
Class I	390	410	430	470	505	535	560	620	640
Master	435	460	485	525	565	595	625	695	715
Elite	480	505	530	575	620	655	685	760	785

(Standards for the 220-pound class were not available as this book was written, but they should be about 370, 435, 525, 590, 660, and 725 for classes IV through Elite.)

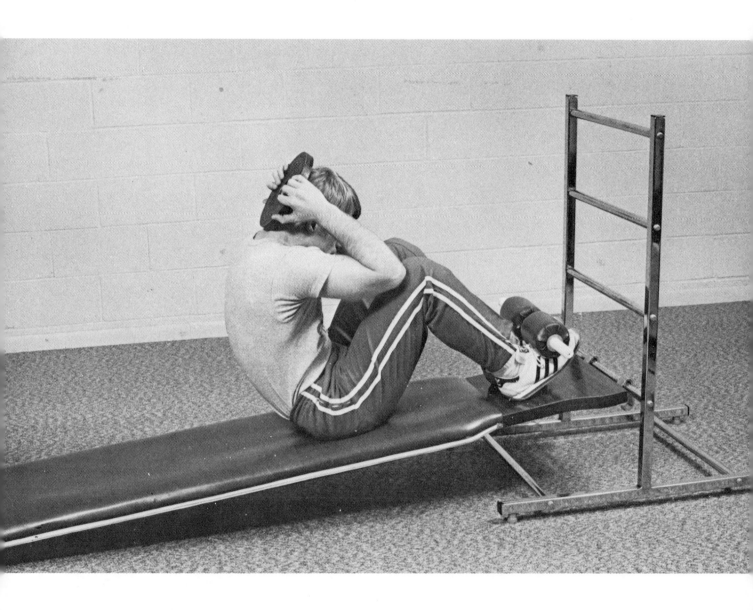

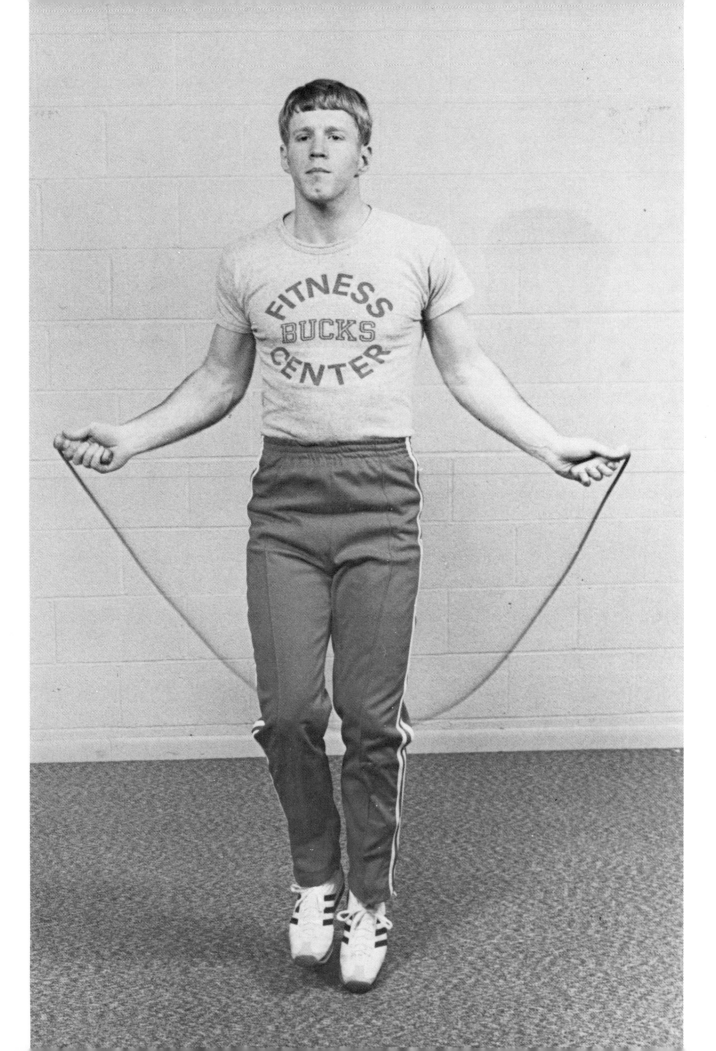

chapter **8**
NUTRITION FOR BUILDING MUSCLE

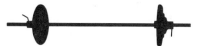

There are unquestionably some strange food fads among athletes and physical culturists. This is frequently pointed out by credentialed experts who do not believe that anyone needs vitamin supplements or large amounts of protein.

The scientific arguments against supplements and other athletic-diet fads are very persuasive, but I would rather look like and be able to perform as well as the faddists than be physically like the credentialed experts.

I am sure, as the experts say, that many of the vitamins ingested by health seekers and would-be champions are excreted to enrich the sewer systems of the nation. But when does the ingestion of such dietary aids pass the point of diminishing returns? It is possible to identify a vitamin deficiency, and it is possible to identify those rare instances of hypervitaminosis that result when someone manages to ingest too much of one of the fat-soluble vitamins, A, D, and K. But who knows what an optimum dose of vitamins is? Some of the recent findings regarding vitamin C suggest that the optimum may be far, far above the minimum requirement needed

to prevent symptoms of deficiency. Therefore it certainly seems prudent for a vigorously active person to supply his or her body with at least a multivitamin supplement to assure that nothing required for optimum performance is missing in an apparently balanced diet.

One bona fide expert who has ample common sense to match his impressive credentials is Jean Mayer, Ph.D., a professor of nutrition who is appropriately skeptical of both "established scientific facts" and the extremes of food faddism. In an interview published in *Family Health* magazine, Dr. Mayer pointed out that "scientific research is changing our ideas all the time. We not only keep learning new things we didn't know before, but we also have to unlearn things we thought we knew, but which now turn out not to be so." He recommends seven groups of foods to obtain the essential nutrients:

1. Leafy green vegetables and yellow vegetables, which provide vitamins (especially vitamin B) and minerals.
2. Citrus fruits, tomatoes, raw cabbage,

and salad greens, which provide vitamin C and roughage.

3. Potatoes and similar root foods as well as fruits to provide starch, vitamins, and minerals.

4. Milk and such milk products as cheese to provide calcium.

5. Meat, poultry, fish, eggs, and legumes for protein and minerals.

6. Bread, flour, and cereals to provide energy, vitamins, iron, and minerals.

7. Butter, margarine, and vegetable oil to provide vitamin A and oil.

Dr. Mayer believes adults should go easy on butter and recommends polyunsaturated margarine, even though—as an unsigned review article in *MD* magazine (March, 1976) points out—"The relationship of dietary cholesterol to total body cholesterol is not scientifically established." Note that Dr. Mayer does not consider sugar a dietary essential. He points out that the body makes its own glucose out of foods in the groups he considers essential. Dr. Mayer does not object to an "occasional" sweet, however.

A major area of disagreement that aligns athletes and their trainers against the nutrition scientists has to do with the body's need for protein. Athletes ingest large amounts of protein foods, including supplements, whereas many academically oriented nutritionists believe that minimum requirements of thirty to forty grams of high quality protein a day are enough. These figures are obtained by allowing seventy milligrams (mg) of nitrogen per kilogram (kg) for a man weighing seventy kg (154 pounds) and then adding thirty percent to provide for individual variations. This level of intake may be safe, but for a man of 175 pounds, 55 gm of protein are required to provide 70 mg of nitrogen per kg, and for a man of 200 pounds, more than 60 gm are required. And the calculations make no allowance for the intense activity of the athlete. Nevin Scrimshaw, Vernon Young, and their associates in the Department of Nutrition and Food Science at the Massachusetts Institute of Technology studied the effect of a diet providing protein at a level equal to the safe practical intake recommended by the 1973 Joint Food and Agriculture Organization Expert Committee on Energy and Protein Requirements. They found that test subjects maintained on this "safe practical intake" suffered decreased lean body and muscle mass, changes in liver metabolism, or both. Obviously such effects would not enhance the performance of an athlete whose sport depends on muscle power. Scrimshaw and Young concluded that "the current recommendations for dietary protein intake for large population groups are inadequate."

On the other hand, protein alone does not meet all the nutritional needs of an athlete. Carbohydrates serve a very important purpose for a person interested in gaining strength and muscular size: they reduce the use of body-building protein for energy. When a person exercises vigorously and consumes a high-protein diet, the expected effect would be an increase in muscle and a decrease in fat, since the body can call upon stored fat more easily than it can on muscle. Once a person is in good shape, however, ingested protein may be used for energy and not for muscle-building if there is an inadequate amount of other energy sources—carbohydrates and fats—in the diet.

Another important point about high-protein diets: It takes about seven times as much water to metabolize protein as it does to metabolize fat or carbohydrate. This is one reason it is important to drink a lot of water while on a diet that is overbalanced on the protein side. To ingest a high-protein diet and simultaneously restrict water intake is asking for kidney trouble.

Just as each individual responds slightly differently to exercise (and should therefore experiment intelligently with training exercises and intensities, and rest periods), so does everyone have to find the diet, with or without supplements, that is best for him or her. People achieve great physical efficiency on many kinds of diets. Some top athletes come from parts of the world where it is hard to obtain the best sources of nutritionally complete protein—eggs, meat, and milk. If wheat bread, which lacks an essential amino acid (lysine), is eaten with cheese, which has the missing amino acid, the mixture provides useful protein. Where even dairy products are in short supply, it is still possible to get enough protein from combinations of beans and rice or rice and peas, which provide mixtures of essential amino acids needed for the protein to be assimilated. In the United States, there are ample supplies of eggs, meat, and dairy products. People who fear the effects of these proteins on their blood cholesterol levels can have these levels monitored medically. That eating eggs and meat will raise cholesterol levels in active people is questionable, however, considering the Masai in Africa, whose chief diet staples are milk and blood. These vigorous herdsmen, who traditionally are prepared to take up spears and defend their cattle against lions, do not seem to have any problems with elevated cholesterol levels.

It appears to be especially important to ingest ample protein during the buildup phase of training. On the other hand, the best time to ingest high-energy "junk" food, such as a candy bar, or a high-carbohydrate meal such as pancakes and syrup, is a few hours before a hard training session or a contest. Incidentally, it takes about four hours after a meal for digestion to progress to the point where you should feel comfortable and perform at your best. A candy bar an hour or less before competition may give you a lift, however. Athletes whose weight is close to the class limit should be cautious about snacks before weigh-ins, but you can gain only six ounces from eating a six-ounce candy bar (providing you don't also drink a few ounces of water!). Some people think they will gain more weight from eating a six-ounce ice cream sundae than from a six-ounce piece of steak. This is not true. When you ingest six ounces, you gain only six ounces. (It is true, however, that over the long-term a high-carbohydrate, sugary sundae is more easily stored as fat than an equal weight of high-protein food.) If you have already made the weight, you may as well obtain the quick energy the sugar provides. The time to build muscle with protein is during the weeks and months of training leading up to the contest.

In general, both common sense and the expertise of people like Dr. Jean Mayer suggest that the real extremes of diet constitute irrational faddism. Dr. Mayer's seven essential nutrients can be recommended as the basis of a balanced diet for anyone in normal health.

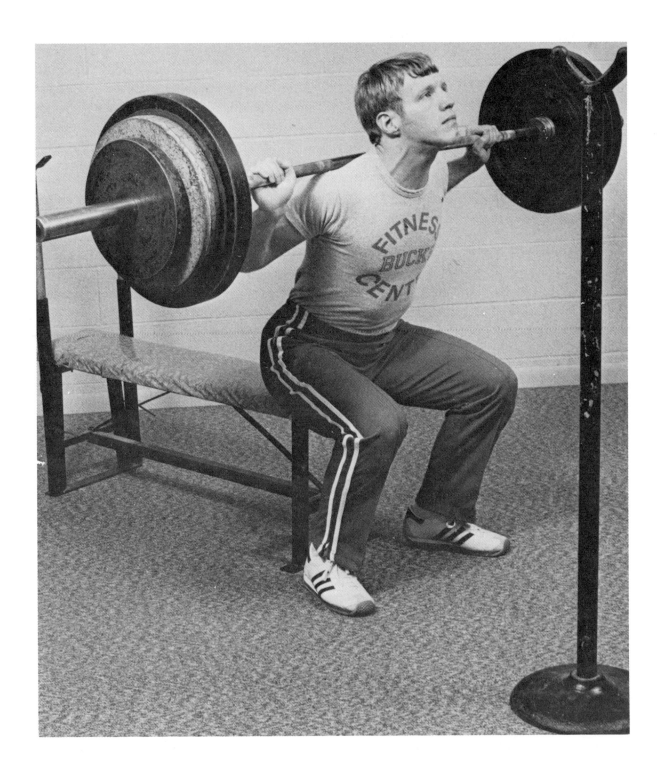

chapter 9
DRUGS AS TRAINING AIDS

One of the most sordid aspects of athletic training and competition is that some ambitious athletes will do anything to gain an advantage over their rivals. This extends to taking drugs that are believed by many to increase energy or to promote muscle size and strength. There are two reasons to object to this practice: (1) If the drug were effective, and the athlete won, he would gain his victory by cheating, since the use of drugs to boost performance violates the rules and spirit of all amateur athletics. Such drug use would be akin to a runner jumping the gun, a thrower surreptitiously using an underweight implement, or a boxer putting a hard object in his glove. (2) No drug effect is gained without paying a price. Even therapeutic drugs must be used with caution, because of their side effects, but when they are given therapeutically there is a trade-off, a balancing of benefits to be received against the hazards of unwanted reactions. The dangerous side effects of such stimulant drugs as amphetamines are well known; there have been a few

deaths of athletes using them in competition. But no one knows the long-term effects of using the anabolic steroids (synthetic male hormones) that athletes take to gain strength and size. The long-term effects of steroids are unknown because these drugs have come into relatively widespread use only in recent years. What we do know, however, is that all steroids have a variety of potent effects and it takes a well-trained, highly skilled physician to use them properly.

A common effect of a steroid drug is to suppress the body's normal production of that steroid. The body in good health has marvelous self-regulating mechanisms, and if you give a hormone to a person whose glands are functioning normally, the body will compensate by reducing its own output of the hormone. An anabolic steroid is an analog of the male hormone testosterone, and if a normal male takes the steroid, there is every reason to expect that his body will reduce its own testosterone output.

Anabolic steroids were developed to help

debilitated, aged people in poor health maintain a positive nitrogen balance. I have not yet heard of any older people given these drugs being sufficiently rejuvenated to win at weight lifting or shot-putting, because despite the best efforts of pharmaceutical chemists and medical scientists, drugs just don't work that miraculously. One reason there are so many different pharmaceutical products for the same indications is that no compound works in exactly the same way in everyone. A skilled physician literally practices the art as well as the science of medicine, learning which medication does the most good for each individual patient. He must do this with great care, always balancing the benefit the patient receives against the possible harm that may be done by a potent compound.

A physician has many useful sources of medical information. One of these is the *Physicians' Desk Reference* (PDR). The PDR indicates that a leading anabolic steroid, one that muscle seekers are reputed to be "munching like peanuts," is only "probably" effective as adjunctive therapy for senile and postmenopausal osteoporosis. The PDR notes that "equal or greater consideration should be given to diet, calcium balance, physiotherapy, and good general health-promoting measures." Under "Warnings," the PDR notes, "Anabolic steroids do not enhance athletic ability." Some of the things a doctor is warned to look out for in patients taking these drugs are these: "Anabolic steroids have been shown to alter glucose tolerance tests.... Since [the drug] contains a 17 alpha alkyl group, liver function should be checked at regular intervals.... Anabolic steroids should be used with caution in patients with benign prostatic hypertrophy.... Serum cholesterol may increase during therapy...."

Adverse reactions that the PDR warns have occurred include "inhibition of testicular function,... oligospermia [deficiency in the number of spermatozoa],... gynecomastia (swollen breasts in males),... inhibition of gonadotropin secretion,... jaundice associated with 17 alpha alkyl substitutions,... decrease in protein bound iodine,... retention of sodium chloride, water, potassium, phosphates, and calcium,... suppression of clotting factors II, V, VII, and X,... decreased 17-ketosteroid excretion...."

If you don't know what those big words mean (and there are more; that's just a sample), you shouldn't be fooling with anabolic steroids, especially in view of the fact that the PDR goes on to note the "proper diet, particularly adequate protein intake, is required to assure the full anabolic benefits of [the drug]." In view of the fact that extensive scientific review has failed to provide positive proof that the drug even does what it was intended to do—help aged people whose own glandular function is subpar—it is quite possible that any athletic improvement that has seemed to come from anabolic drugs may have resulted from a combination of good nutrition and hard training, boosted by the athlete's expectation of positive results (the "placebo effect"). The mind can play many tricks, and it may enable an athlete to progress in spite of anabolics as well as because of them.

Contrast the careful practice of therapeutic medicine, with monitoring of liver function and so forth, with the uncontrolled pill gulping that is reputed to go on among would-be champion athletes. What does the athlete know of inhibited gonadotropin secretion? Of long-term liver damage? Of the painful death that can result from prostatic cancer?

But, you may wonder, what if the Eastern Europeans are taking these drugs? If they are, one must hope for their sakes that the medical supervision is adequate to protect them against all the possible long-term adverse effects that can result from tampering with the superb functioning of a naturally superior body.

I am not making any attempt to review the scientific literature on anabolic steroids in this book, or even to present a balanced discussion. My main reason for taking an antidrug stand—aside from the moral issue—is that I don't believe there is nearly enough evidence available on the long-term effects of these compounds for anyone to comment definitively on their safety or efficacy. I have seen reports on apparently well-controlled and carefully conducted scientific studies that indicate that anabolic steroids have no appreciable effect on strength. Other studies suggest that the drugs may boost strength, and a number of people whose opinions I respect are convinced that weight lifters are reaching new heights—not without a variety of physical costs—as a result of taking them.

Personally, I believe that progress in athletic achievement would have proceeded at the same pace without the drugs. No one has yet developed anything in a test tube that will make a champion out of a duffer. There have been improvements in training methods, equipment, technique, and nutrition. In the case of the European athletes, there has been a concerted talent search to find the young people with the potential to become champions. In the United States, people are free to find their own way, and many of the most athletically gifted young people choose to participate in sports that will later enable them to earn good livings as professionals; they opt for baseball or football rather than such Olympic sports as track or wrestling or weight lifting. There are many things for young Americans to do, and there may be potential Olympic champions who prefer to study or listen to music rather than take part in sports, though it is doubtful that many champions are lost in this way. But I do believe the interaction of these many factors has more to do with the success of Europe's "amateur" athletes than any magic pill or injection. And I urge young athletes to participate in sports for the fun and sense of achievement that they can gain from them naturally, without depending on the psychological or chemical boost that they might possibly obtain from drugs. If they can win without cheating, victory will be sweeter. If their athletic training and participation carries over into vigorous and disease-free later lives, the reward will be truly worthwhile.

REFERENCES

Although this publication is an instruction manual rather than a textbook, some readers may be interested in reading some of the source material used.

ON THE PHYSIOLOGY OF EXERCISE

Faria, I. E. 1970. Cardiovascular response to exercise as influenced by training of various intensities. *Research Quarterly,* 41: 44–50.

Fox, E. L., 1973. Intensity and distance of interval training programs and changes in aerobic power. *Medicine and Science in Sports* 5: 18–22.

Gordon, E. E. 1967. Anatomical and biochemical adaptations of muscle to different exercises. *Journal of the American Medical Association* 201: 129–32.

Gordon, E. E., 1967. Adaptations of muscle to various exercises. *Journal of the American Medical Association* 199: 139–44.

Karpovich, P. V. 1959. *Physiology of Muscular Activity.* Philadelphia: W. B. Saunders Co.

Paffenbarger, R. S., and Hale, W. E. 1975. Work activity and coronary heart mortality. *New England Journal of Medicine* 292: 545–50.

Rasch, P. J., and Burke, R. K. 1963. *Kinesiology and Applied Anatomy.* Philadelphia: Lea & Febiger.

Zohman, L. R. 1974. *Exercise Your Way to Fitness and Heart Health.* C.P.C. International.

ON WEIGHT LIFTING AND WEIGHT TRAINING

Abbo, F. E. 1966. Weight lifting held to raise steroids to "youthful" levels. *Medical Tribune,* May 4, 1966, p. 29.

Howell, M. L., and Morford, W. R. 1964. Circuit training for a college fitness program. *Journal of Health, Physical Education and Recreation,* February 1964, pp. 30, 31, 72.

Iron Man magazine. 1950–1977. Alliance, Neb.

Murray, J., and Karpovich, P. V. 1956. *Weight Training in Athletics.* Englewood Cliffs, N. J.: Prentice-Hall.

Muscle Builder/Power magazine. 1960–1977. Woodland Hills, Calif.

Nagy, George, ed. 1974–1975. *Weight Lifting Handbook.* Indianapolis: Amateur Athletic Union of the United States.

Strength & Health magazine. 1940–1977. York, Pa.

Willoughby, D. P. 1970. *The Super Athletes.* Cranbury, N. J.: A. S. Barnes & Co.

ON NUTRITION

Engel, M. J., and Rudolph, M. 1970. Let's talk about good foods: A conversation with Prof. Jean Mayer. *Family Health,* July 1970, pp. 26–29.

MD magazine (special issue on nutrition). March 1976, pp. 100–111.

Scrimshaw, N. S., and Young, V. R. 1976. The requirements of human nutrition. *Scientific American* 235: 51–64.

ON DRUGS IN SPORTS

Cooper, D. L. 1972. Drugs and the athlete. *Journal of the American Medical Association.* 221: 1007–11.

Golding, L. A., *et al:* 1974. Weight, size and strength—unchanged with steroids. *Physician and Sportsmedicine* 2: 39–43.

Physicians' Desk Reference. 1976. Sections on anabolic steroids. Oradell, N. J.: Medical Economics.

Wade, N. 1972. Anabolic steroids: Doctors denounce them but athletes aren't listening. *Science* 176: 1399–1403.

index